BIPOLAR

HAS

1000

FACES

PSYCHIATRY ENLIGHTENMENT
Shreveport, Louisiana

Interior Design: J. L. Saloff
Cover Design: Mark Saloff Designs

Copyright information available upon request. v. 3

Print ISBN: 978-0-9962701-2-0
E-book ISBN: 978-0-9962701-3-7
Library of Congress Number: 2019908457
First Edition © 2015

Published in the United States of America on acid-free paper.

Third Edition

"Making Diagnosis Simple"

BIPOLAR
HAS
1000
FACES

Jesse Lee Hite, M.D.

PSYCHIATRY ENLIGHTENMENT

TABLE OF CONTENTS

DISCLAIMER

The author does not assume responsibility for the mental or physical health of any reader or anyone who obtains this information from a reader. Each reader is responsible for carefully selecting their personal physicians who are medicolegally responsible for their health within the limits of applicable law. This book contains the opinions of the author. It is solely for informational and educational purposes. It was never intended to substitute for professional medical treatment. Neither the author or anyone associated with publishing this book will be responsible or liable for loss or damage allegedly arising from any opinion or information in this book.

To my patients who taught me all I know.

INTRODUCTION

I am writing this book for the third time. I first wrote it in 2015 when I was at the peak of my knowledge. I wrote each chapter over and over. One goal was to make it grammatically perfect. Another goal was to make each description of mental illness as simple as possible so that people without a medical background could easily understand it. Then I revised several chapters in 2019 because of new knowledge or new experiences. But how to make a book of knowledge interesting? That is why I'm writing this book for the third time. I hope to make it more interesting. Jesus taught in parables. I wish I could do that. Perhaps you should read a chapter now and then. Each chapter is full of knowledge, very worthwhile, practically no fluff. This can be very tiring. I'm sorry. In spite of all my efforts, it would probably be more beneficial if you read a chapter now and then—no attempt to read it all at once.

One of the most important things I will discuss in this book is "Mixed Mania." I listen carefully to academic leaders in psychiatry. I respectfully attend their lectures. Honestly, I think busy psychiatrists who see many, many patients know more about the many facets of psychiatry than do the professors they are so respectfully listening to. But, lecturers in high academic standing have more power than other psychiatrists. People listen to power. I have made many efforts to submit a letter, not a high-powered double-blind, randomized, controlled study with two pages of statistics, peer-reviewed (probably academic friends) etc. I am hoping someone who has the ability to do this type of research will be motivated by my simple letter to do so. So far, none of the journals have even responded to me. That happens a lot these days. They don't see anything in it for them in terms of increasing their prestige or their salary. Actually, they are wrong about this. "Mixed Mania" is unbelievably common and usually the diagnosis is missed.

A mother brings her 16-year-old daughter in for our first consultation. Her grades in school indicate that she is very bright. She has made six suicidal attempts and has been hospitalized four times in the last two years of her short life. She has seen several different psychiatrists and she has been treated with several different antidepressants—all to no avail. That story pricks my ears up right away. A classical presentation of mixed mania. I ask her two simple questions. "How many hours does it take you to fall asleep at night?" The answer is usually five or six hours. This is a symptom of mania—not depression. Second question, "Is your mind racing?" This is a hard question for many patients, but not if they have mixed mania. Their answer will come quickly and without hesitation. This is a second symptom of mania, not depression. They do not have the third prominent symptom of classical mania which is highly increased energy causing them to drive 120 mph down the highway, drink more, eat more, have more sex, etc. This third symptom of mania can take many forms. I will discuss this more in later chapters. Mania can have many different affects, like extreme euphoria, rage, etc. But this 16-year-old girl did not have any of these manifestations of extreme increase in energy. She looked depressed. She talked about depression. She did not look manic at all. That diagnosis had not even been considered by her previous psychiatrists. She just looked depressed. But, she exhibited two symptoms of mania in addition to her depression. Her depression went into remission when I gave her low dosages of medications for mania while gradually discontinuing her medications for depression, which never work for this problem. This is an unusually simple case, but I used it to get my point across. The mother worked in retail. I saw her about one and a half years later. Her daughter no longer took a mood stabilizer, but she quickly turned to the Risperdal I had prescribed, low dosage, whenever her difficulty with sleep or depression recurred. She had not been seriously depressed in the last 18 months or so. Probably, she was being treated by her family physician.

About three years later, I was working at our local VA hospital. A 29-year-old female came to my office for her first interview. She immediately told me that she had mixed mania. You can imagine that I was surprised at her knowledge of her diagnosis. I ask her how she knew? She was hospitalized at a local private hospital because the inpatient unit at the VA was full. She was treated by a very busy psychiatrist (not a major academician.) I believe a very busy psychiatrist sees many more patients than the most prestigious academicians who spend so much time doing sophisticated research, writing papers, lecturing, etc. Psychiatric diagnosis is learned only by seeing a lot of patients. This psychiatrist had discontinued her antidepressants and prescribed low dosages of medications for mania. Her depression (mixed mania) was much improved. All I had to do was continue the same medications. She had been on antidepressants for 17 years, since age 12. (Notice that I dedicated this book to my patients "who taught me all I know.")

Addition: I just reviewed the medical records of some of my patients whom I saw in my first 15 years of private practice. In reading their initial interview and past history, it looks as though I might have missed the diagnosis on several of them. I did not become a good diagnostician during those first 15 years. Psychiatric residencies today are better than mine, 1959-1962. But I still believe these young psychiatrists will need to see quite a number of patients before they become good diagnosticians.

MY JOURNEY TO UNDERSTANDING

I went to medical school at the University of Texas—Medical Branch in the 1950s. I had a rotating internship at Hermann Hospital in Houston, Texas. My residency in psychiatry between 1959 and 1962 was at the VA hospital in Topeka, Kansas strongly affiliated with the Menninger School of Psychiatry which was dominated at that time by psychoanalysts. Most of the departments of psychiatry in well-known universities around the country were dominated by psychoanalysts. That was not entirely true across the South. The new medications to treat mental illness were just being developed by a Dr. Janssen. I'm not positive, but I believe he was affiliated with Roche Pharmaceuticals.

I became acquainted with schizophrenic patients who had become ill during the second world war. Due to the new medications, patients this ill are rarely seen today. They had been in the hospital for at least 15 years, and it looked as if they would be there for the rest of their lives. Fortunately, I was also introduced to acute mental illness which could frequently be treated with the new medications. I treated my first schizophrenic patient with a very new medication called Stelazine. To my amazement, his auditory hallucinations, delusional thinking etc. cleared rather rapidly. I discharged him to his home in Tulsa, Oklahoma. Within a couple of months he was back in the hospital with me as his physician. He was a veteran with a significant amount of cash. The voices told him to go out on a hillside and commit "Hari Kari." As he plunged the knife into his belly, he came to his senses and drove to the nearest emergency room. I gave him the same medications, and he responded again. I have no follow-up on him beyond that point. Schizophrenic patients often develop some "insight" after these experiences. Sometimes they even come to realize that other people don't hear the voices they hear and that other people don't see the visual hallucinations that they see. I spent six months on a neurological ward. I spent one and a half years doing psychotherapy with supervision. The total time was three years. Today, many residents spend up to five or six years to become accredited as child psychiatrist or other disciplines.

In those days there was a draft. I was immediately sent to Tachikawa, Japan to join four other psychiatrist who took care of the Far East including places like the Philippines, Okinawa, etc. I was newly married. The war in Vietnam had not yet started. Technically, I am a veteran, but I don't feel like one because I had such a wonderful assignment in Japan during peacetime. One of my patients, waiting to be shipped back to the United States for more extensive treatment, saved his sleep medication (Dalmane) for several weeks, I don't know exactly how long. One night, he took them all. The next morning he did not get up for roll call. He slept for five days. He awoke very unhappy that his suicidal attempt had failed. Notice that this terrible, old, long-lasting benzodiazepine did not kill him. It would have if it were mixed with other sedatives. Benzodiazepines alone usually do not kill people. Later in the book I've written a chapter entitled "Addressing the Prejudice Against Benzodiazepines."

I can't say why, but for some reason I was eager to get out of the Air Force and return to the United States to start my private practice. I had traveled across the country and seen California, the coast, for the first time. I had flown in a plane for the first time. After driving up and down the coast, amazed by the wonderful temperature in the summer, I took a job in San Diego for six months in charge of the female ward at the local County Hospital. For reasons that are quite obscure, I ended up starting my first private practice on Palos Verdes Peninsula. Friends I met in Japan helped me to get it started. I also worked downtown Los Angeles with San Quentin parolees. I borrowed $2000 from the Hong Kong–Shanghai Bank in downtown Los Angeles to live on. Four years later, I moved to Santa Rosa, California to help open the first psychiatric hospital in Sonoma County. Santa Rosa had a population of 45,000. Drinks at the local bar were $0.25. After nine months, I returned to Los Angeles. I am not going to tell you about all the different places I have worked. Winston Churchill said that "Success is going from failure to failure with enthusiasm." In my case, I stumbled from failure to failure with bouts of anxiety and depression.

From 1980 to 1994 I practiced anesthesia including the initial two-year residency. After that, I returned to the practice of psychiatry in my present location, Shreveport, Louisiana. Here I have worked in private hospitals, private outpatient, mental health clinics in Shreveport and Monroe Louisiana, often treating children as well as adults. I estimate that I have 13 years experience treating children. I also ran a geriatric unit for at least 18 months. I worked at the local VA. Then after 2015, I went to certain institutions in Texas for short assignments working with the intellectually disabled. I saw many illnesses there that I had never seen before. This type of work is called *locum tenens*, and the assignments are usually about three months to one year. The last 6 months was spent working with intellectually disabled felons ages 18 to 30. Over 45 years, I have heard about many horrible childhoods. But, the stories I heard working with these young intellectually disabled felons were the worst I have ever heard. One young man observed his father having sex with his sister. Being intellectually disabled, he tried the same thing. He ended up in court as a felon. As I stated earlier, I stumbled from experience to experience with bouts of anxiety and depression. I forgot to mention that I did teach psychiatry in a good department for a few months and I taught anesthesia for three years.

Chapter 1

THE INNER CRITIC

*"I have noticed my conscience for many years,
and I know it is more trouble and bother to me than
anything else I started with." ~Mark Twain*

Obviously, Mark Twain was an introspective author. One of my critic's stated that the inner critic is nothing more than one's conscience. Well, maybe so, but each of us has a conscience that is extremely different from one person to another. And frequently, our conscience is an extremely severe inner critic. I got the name "Inner Critic" from a psychoanalyst, Louis Paul, MD, in Beverly Hills around the late 1960s or early 1970s. I would drive 45 minutes up the coast to see him, during my first private practice, to help me with my more difficult patients in psychotherapy. He was a genius at seeing the workings of the inner critic in my patients, some of whom were rather mysterious to me as to what their basic problem was. The inner critic is a problem which can be successfully worked with, overtime, in psychotherapy if the patient is not severely mentally ill.

Throughout most of my career, I have dealt with serious mental illness. These illnesses required medication. Schizophrenia cannot be treated successfully without the use of medication. Serious bipolar disorder requires medication. Psychotherapy may be a modifying factor if these illnesses are of a mild nature. Many patients become addicted to their psychotherapist. Sometimes I was giving a severely ill patient medication which was essential to keep her from committing suicide or ending up in jail, etc. But on occasion, I have had a patient of this nature who would miss an appointment with me, but never miss an appointment with their therapist.

Many severely ill schizophrenic patients have a horrible inner critic. But, the inner critic is more obvious in bipolar patients. During mania their inner critic is extremely muted. They are proud of themselves. They like to be seen. They may wear bright colored clothes. They talk freely to everyone. Actually, their affect can vary from euphoria to rage; so my description above is primarily of the classically euphoric manic. Also this is a very obvious manic. They are not always so obvious. I had one veteran at the VA hospital who was shoplifting fairly routinely. He did not think he would get caught. He always had a sly smile on his face. His diminished inner critic was not so obvious to others. Actually, he had been caught several times. The judge promised to send him to prison if he continued. On initial meeting, one would not recognize his mania until he told you his feelings and his circumstances. But there was a greatly diminished inner critic whether it was obvious or not. I had a young felon, age 23, in an institution for intellectually disabled felons, who stole one cellphone each month just to keep in practice. He was a quiet person, but he always had a sly smile. He was not uncomfortable when I discussed his problem with the treatment group when he was manic. Later, when he was depressed (stronger inner critic) he would become very uncomfortable when confronted with this problem, obviously embarrassed.

The bipolar patient, during episodes of depression, have a very severe inner critic. They avoid people. They do not talk very much. Men in positions of authority wear dark gray suits only, no uninhibited behavior or bright clothes. Here, I am referring to a schoolteacher I knew. When I first met him, he was dressed in a dark gray suit, very depressed. The very next appointment he had rotated into mania. He was wearing a yellow sport coat and orange pants. He was very jolly. He actually got into some trouble for taking money from a prohibited fund to throw a party for the students of the school. The inner critic was greatly diminished while he was manic, and his judgment was diminished.

People with a strong inner critic, but not overwhelmed

by it, are sometimes referred to as the "salt of the earth." The philosopher Kant spoke of the "good will" as being like a diamond. It is of great value whether the human being is very intelligent or not so intelligent. People with a strong inner critic might not be too successful in business. After all, to make money you have to take it away from somebody. Someone with a strong inner critic would have trouble being a successful politician. A successful politician has to tell each big donor what they want to hear. They must not be too bothered by the truth to respond in a sincere and convincing manner. I want my plumber to have the goodwill. The same for my electrician, etc. But one surgeon told me that the only surgeons who do not have mishaps are the ones who never operate. I want my surgeon to have a reasonable inner critic, the goodwill, but I do not want him to be destroyed by his inner critic with every surgical mishap. His ability as a surgeon would be greatly diminished.

The majority of mentally ill people have a severe inner critic. I rarely have a narcissistic patient. I have known several brilliant, accomplished narcissistic people, but by definition they do not have much empathy for lesser human beings. They can see the workings of the inner critic in people around them. They will frequently use their inner critic to manipulate them into doing something for others (usually profitable to the narcissistic person) but not in the best interest of their victim. Sometimes if attacked, the narcissistic person will use the inner critic of their attacker to demolish their self-esteem. I have on occasion had this happen to me while in a subjugated position during years of learning to become a physician. It is very important for each one of us to recognize this maneuver and protect our self-esteem from these narcissistic people. As I mentioned earlier, they do not have much empathy for "lesser human beings." They attack when you have said something, almost anything, that might diminish their usually overinflated self-esteem. They do not tolerate criticism unless they are in an inferior position of power. They may then say things to inflate the ego of their direct superiors.

Most people are only aware of a portion of their inner critic. This is where a good psychotherapist can be of value if their inner critic is unrealistically severe. Everything the patient tells you, no matter what they are talking about, reveals their inner critic to an experienced psychotherapist. The psychotherapist becomes extremely sensitive to the workings of the inner critic in their patient no matter what the misery was that brought them to see the therapist. Helping the patient reason against their unrealistic inner critic takes time. First the patient must become aware more and more of the workings of their inner critic. How can the patient reason against something they are not aware of. This may take many sessions of psychotherapy as the patient gradually becomes more and more aware of their inner critic. Then the patient must practice reasoning against their inner critic while they are not under the guidance of their therapist.

Neuroscientist have reasons to believe that the bulk of the inner critic resides in the brain just above the bony orbits around your eyes. This is called the orbitofrontal cortex. Above that lies the dorsolateral prefrontal cortex. Superior reasoning occurs in the dorsolateral prefrontal cortex. In the past, during psychotherapy, I can almost imagine myself reasoning with the patient's dorsolateral prefrontal cortex against their overdeveloped, powerful, orbitofrontal cortex. If a human being or an animal sustains damage to the orbitofrontal cortex, it will have a dramatic effect on their personality. Animals will not take the trouble to nurture their offspring. People are similar. A very disciplined and moral human being can change dramatically after damage to the orbitofrontal cortex.

During serious mental illness, the patient may begin to hear voices telling him that he is worthless. Many depressed patients, even if they're not hearing voices, tell me that they feel worthless. If they are sick enough, the inner critic will reason with them, often through voices, that they should commit suicide. They will make it sound like the logical thing to do. The patient may have difficulty using their reason to avoid suicide. This is not meant to be any sort of a comprehensive discussion of suicide. Suicide occurs for many reasons not mentioned here. But suicide is very frequent in bipolar patients, especially when they are in a profound depression. Auditory hallucinations do occur in very serious bipolar disorder.

They can occur during mania and during depression. As you would expect, their messages to the patient vary greatly between depression and mania. Schizophrenic patients usually hear voices. Everyone knows this. Sometimes a severely ill bipolar patient hearing voices can appear to be schizophrenic. But if the psychiatrist knows the past history of the patient, he will be able to differentiate between schizophrenia and severe bipolar disorder. Sometimes there is a never-ceasing overlap between these two illnesses, and the patient will receive a diagnosis of schizoaffective disorder.

A very severe inner critic in a supposedly normal person can lead to greatly diminished self-esteem and low-grade depression which may never receive treatment. The person is so accustomed to this state of mind that they do not realize their condition. During a few moments of happiness with increased self-esteem and diminished inner critic they may develop some insight. They might or might not qualify for psychotherapy or antidepressant treatment. They might seek treatment depending on how miserable they are. This is not an unusual condition. A few people are very fortunate in that they are always in a state of very mild mania with a somewhat diminished inner critic. They may be very productive in multiple different ways depending on their talents. Some may be motivational speakers for the less fortunate, or painters, or authors, or industrialist depending on their interest and talents. This type of person could be very successful in business ventures. They also have increased energy to succeed at whatever they might try. Remember, Winston Churchill said that success was going from failure to failure with enthusiasm. These people are not often depressed.

When people take a few drinks of alcohol, or a few puffs of marijuana, or any other "feel-good drug" they become quite happy sometimes referred to as a "high." This feeling is due to an increased amount of the neurotransmitter dopamine. In some way, dopamine must diminish the power of the inner critic. They are relieved from self-doubt and anxieties. They do not worry about what other people think of them. I have heard it said that alcohol is a social lubricant.

People are in better control of their inner critic when they are in their best condition physically. When they are tired, the inner critic may be more powerful. Their power of reasoning is diminished. People can be unrealistically guilty about many things.

Just as the inner critic may interfere with business judgment, it may also interfere with personal judgments concerning marriage, etc. It may be very difficult to terminate a relationship with a good person who just happens to be in love with you. Obviously, you would not terminate the relationship if your feelings for the other person were similar. Even then, for some reason you may know that you should not marry that person. The inner critic can play havoc in your judgment during the very exciting times of dating and partner selection.

The origins of the inner critic are complex and beyond the scope of this chapter. Nature or nurture. How much depends upon parenting. How much depends upon inheritance. The latter would also be called genetics.

Since the inner critic changes with almost every facet of mental illness, this discussion could go on and on. Perhaps this is a good place to stop, but the subject matter is not exhausted.

But wait, I have one last story to tell. I will never forget two brothers in their early 20s that I met many years ago. The conscientious brother was studying to become a physician. He was just about to enter medical school. During the summer he took a trip with his father to Italy. He developed severe paranoid schizophrenia. When I first met him in a psychiatric unit, he was sitting up in bed trying to eat soup with a fork. He was still partially restrained. He recovered well and entered medical school, but I do not have any follow-up as to how he performed. His brother had curly black hair, a flashing beautiful smile, never had much guilt, and was leading a happy, self-fulfilling life. I have noticed that one young man will go to church and feel compelled to become a missionary.

Another young man will attend the same church. The thought of becoming a missionary never crosses his mind.

Chapter 2

Bipolar I Disorder

Bipolar I disorder is composed of two poles which I will describe as the "*Speeded up Pole*" and the "*Slowed Down Pole*." Bipolar I can be in either pole for long periods of time. Bipolar II is characterized by long serious depressions with only a few days, not very often, of mania. Bipolar II depression is different from the *slowed down pole* (depression) of Bipolar I disorder. The treatment is quite different. So I am making the description of bipolar II depression in a separate chapter to follow.

Speeded Up Pole

First, let's discuss the *Speeded up Pole* of Bipolar I Disorder. So, mania presents with many faces. But all three presentations exhibit an extreme increase in energy with a racing mind and difficulty falling asleep. Mixed mania will have the racing mind and difficulty falling asleep, but not the very high energy level. Classical Bipolar I Mania does not present as depressed to the best of my recollections.

The increased energy of the Bipolar I illness is usually easily observed, sometimes more obvious than others. This diagnosis is rarely missed.

The *speeded up pole* of Bipolar I disorder is like an actress on a stage. Dramatic. Causes a lot of attention. As you know, a good actress can carry a stage play or a movie. A good actress is almost essential to a successful movie. The *speeded up pole* is like a good actress; these people attract attention. Consequently straightforward Bipolar I mania is rarely misdiagnosed. They can be happy or enraged with everyone, or extremely physically active, but they stand out like a "sore thumb" because of their greatly increased energy level. The happy ones are usually very verbose and very animated in their speech. They are thinking and talking fast. I had one bright, highly-animated patient who could tell me three jokes before I could ask my first question. Then he would answer my questions before I could complete the question. He could not help reading my mind to some extent. Very bright, very quick of thought, very quick of speech. At times, he would exhibit "a flight of ideas." His speech would go from topic to topic to topic — all totally disconnected as best I could tell. A "flight of ideas" is classic for the happy manic. This is a fairly serious mania.

Some people have a very mild mania, called hypomania, which is beneficial in their work, particularly if they are in sales or an inspirational speaker for example. People with hypomania are experiencing no pain mentally, and do not seek help.

The classic manic loses the normal self-consciousness that most of us have. He or she is absolutely sure of themselves — the opposite of depression where making a decision is so difficult. Without self-consciousness, they dress in a more dramatic way be they male or female. I had one very modest female patient who would put on a flimsy purple dress and dance in a provocative manner after admission to the psychiatric unit. After treatment and discharge, she came to my office with her daughter dressed very modestly. Note the change of personality.

Most mental illness, be it bipolar disorder or schizophrenia or some other mental illness, is usually heralded by a definite change of personality. So, among your friends and relatives, watch for sudden, often dramatic, changes of personality. They may be slipping into a mental illness. Due to this dramatic decrease in the inner critic (explained in an earlier chapter), which eliminates self-consciousness, they may participate in extramarital affairs. They can consume more alcohol, eat more food, drive long distances often at high speeds, need larger doses of medication, start new businesses which are probably doomed to failure, etc. etc. They feel so good that they may not want treatment. They may sleep only two or three hours per night, but they may never feel tired.

I had one patient who thought he was "Elvis." He

went up and down the hall of the psychiatric unit singing at the top of his lungs. The nursing staff hid themselves in their offices. The other patients were hiding under their beds. He would then ask me "Why won't nobody talk to me?" It took me over 52 days to "bring him down." The amount of various medications that I gave him would cause criticism from most other psychiatrists. But if they were in my shoes, they would have done something similar. Actually, I transferred him to another psychiatrist in another hospital who increased his Depakote to a level which would be considered malpractice. He went home, went into a coma, and when he awoke, the mania was gone. Sometimes these very serious manic patients are treated successfully with electric shock treatment. I think his reaction to the high dose of Depakote, which affected his brain adversely, cured his mania. Severe mania can be very difficult to treat.

The enraged, angry, severe manics also have a high level of energy. But they don't feel so good. They would like to feel different, but they can't. They are sure of themselves. They may or may not accept treatment. They often lose their job after they verbally berate their employers. They scream at their relatives. They scream at their friends who may no longer be friendly. Their judgment is very flawed like the happy manic. They can only sleep two or three hours per night. Their speech is rapid, but their rage is more noticeable. I will never forget an older, white-haired woman who was verbally pecking on her husband's head like two birds. Her rage was obvious and never-ending.

A few severe manics will take on a weightlifting program, train for a marathon, etc. Often they have never done anything like this in the past — note the change in personality — keep your eyes open for the change of personality. Everyone thought this young man was improving his lifestyle.

I mentioned earlier the three most common types of mania. One of them was the one who exhibits a greatly increased energy level manifested physically, primarily. I had one housewife who built a new porch for her house. She had never done anything like this before — personality change. I had one housewife who used her energy to scrub the grout in her bathroom with a toothbrush.

Of course, like other patients with mania, they can only sleep a couple of hours per night. These women are in sharp contrast to the women who go to a local bar, drink quite a bit of alcohol, and have a one night stand. They are both manic, but superficially very different. Mania has a thousand faces.

Sometimes they begin to hear voices praising them for their many outstanding qualities. When reality becomes extremely distorted, we call it psychosis. Manics can become psychotic hearing voices, etc.

Sometimes these people are so psychotic as to resemble schizophrenia. If a new psychiatrist inherited this patient without seeing the gradual worsening of mania into psychosis, he might have a difficult time deciding whether the diagnosis was schizophrenia or psychotic mania. Sometimes they have symptoms diagnostic of mania and schizophrenia so that they receive a diagnosis of Schizoaffective disorder. Then they will receive treatment for both illnesses at the same time. There is considerable overlap in medications for treatment of bipolar mania and schizophrenia anyway.

Remember, extremely mild mania can be advantageous for painting great paintings or writing great books or selling ideas or things to other people. But this is very mild mania. The psychiatric textbooks used to estimate severe mania as 1% of the population. Schizophrenia was also 1% of the population. More recently, due to greater diagnostic sensitivity, that figure has been raised to 7% for severe mania. Actually, mood disorders probably affect at least 25 to 30% of our population. Recently I have read even higher percentages? Why do you think so many marriages fail? Unrecognized mood disorders lead to divorce, dropping out of college, and many other unfortunate happenings.

They also lead to suicide. I have known several patients and several physicians who committed suicide to my great surprise. I have known two male patients who committed suicide after having trouble finding work for several years. These suicides are more understandable and somewhat more predictable, but most of the suicides I have experienced were completely unpredictable. The person did not share their plan with anyone. The last physician I knew to do this was, in my mind, the best-adjusted man and psychiatrist I had ever met. I had him on a pedestal. He hung himself from one of the rafters in his living room. His wife was understandably heartbroken.

As a footnote, many of these people become addicted to alcohol or use marijuana to excess. What would you do if you could never get over three hours sleep per night and your mind was constantly racing? You would look for relief somehow. You might not recognize that you are mentally ill and need psychiatric help. This illness is a frequent road to addiction.

Slowed Down Pole

This depression is not so different from the classical depression I attempt to describe in another chapter. And, fortunately, it will respond to antidepressants, mood stabilizers, etc. Frequently it is difficult to distinguish this bipolar depression from a classical depression. The past history is very helpful. If they have ever had an episode of mania, then the diagnosis becomes more obvious. A good history of previous mania may be hard to obtain. The episode could be classical mania or maybe a mania of short duration. It may be difficult to decide if the mood change of short duration was really mania or not. This history is taken in the context of trying to decide if this episode of depression is classical depression or bipolar depression. They do not have prominent symptoms of insomnia or a racing mind like mixed mania. Even though antidepressants are essential in treatment, these patients also need mood stabilizers, perhaps like lithium as an example. In the past few years, there has been a great deal of talk among psychiatrists as to the safety of administering antidepressants to these patients. There has been a concern that the antidepressants might cause a "flip" back into mania. That is one reason to give mood stabilizers. You can see that the treatment for this type of depression is somewhat different from the treatment for a classical depression.

How do I play it? If the patient has a past history of horrible mania where no one could keep him from driving 120 mph. If the patient has had frequent episodes of mania (*speeded up pole*) and rare episodes of the (*slowed down pole*). If his depressions are of short duration. In other words, he is much more prone to mania than depression. Considering this past history, I might not treat the depression aggressively for fear of flipping him back into mania. He may have to just live through the depression, assuming he will soon be manic again. But, usually, I can treat the depression aggressively without causing mania.

In the past, I was treating an elderly female for bipolar disorder. Her memory was changing slightly. She always called me, about once every two weeks, in a state of severe depression. I assumed that the depression was her main problem. But, fortunately, a caretaker began a diary of her mood swings. The diary revealed that she was manic all the time, except when she called me for treatment of depression. These depressions only lasted two or three days. The rest of the time she was manic. She liked her episodes of mania and did not bother to phone me. Except for the diary, I would have been giving her antidepressants which probably would have made her mania worse. I did not attempt to treat these brief episodes of depression.

I had an adolescent, age 14, who would be manic with the racing mind and severe rage for about four days, then he would be perfectly normal for about four days. Notice the extreme difference between this patient and the one who thought he was "Elvis." In one patient the mania went on and on. In this adolescent, the mania only lasted four days. During those four days, his behavior in school was intolerable. He was expelled over and over. Then he would be perfectly normal for four days. By the time I met him he was permanently expelled from the public school. These last two examples would probably be defined as "rapid cycling."

I recently saw a show on television concerning a young woman shooting a young man who was rejecting her romantically. He was not steadfast in the rejection but frequently changed his mind rotating his affections back and forth between two women. He had a gun in every room of his house. She had texted him 50 times that day. Do you see "increased energy?" When she went to his house that evening, he was again partially responsive to her romantically. During an argument, she grabbed for a gun lying on the table between them. She shot him fatally. During the interrogation at the police station, she rapidly admitted her guilt. She did not lie to create an impression of self-defense, although it may have been in self-defense. Notice her lack of judgment in her self-defense. When the examiner walked out of the room, she was walking around the room saying over and over, "Yep, I did it. Yep, I did it." She even did a twirl or two as she walked around the room. The police were watching her through a one-way mirror. They thought her behavior was proof that she was the killer and without any remorse. My opinion is that she was manic. Note the increased energy. Note the lack of remorse, which is classical for mania because of their decrease in the "inner critic."

Walking around the room like that, with an occasional twirl, is not normal when you're looking at life in prison. Texting 50 times in one day is crazy. I think she was manic. Her mug shot showed her to be very wide-eyed and wired in general. She received 40 years in prison. Later at a retrial, due to some infraction of the rules in the first trial, her facial expressions were perfectly normal. She did not look "bug-eyed." Her behavior was perfectly normal. I do not believe she was manic at that time. So, she received a 100-year sentence at the second trial. I would like to know what her behavior was like in jail during the six years between the trials. Did she have many marked changes in personality perhaps indicating bipolar disorder? This story indicates the many subtleties of bipolar disorder. The diagnoses can be obvious sometimes, but the diagnoses can be very puzzling at other times. She was evaluated by two psychiatrists who testified in court. Neither one even mentioned the possibility of bipolar mania.

Chapter 3

BIPOLAR II DISORDER

This depression is quite different from the Bipolar I depression I was just describing. They have usually had extremely brief episodes of mania hardly worth mentioning. Otherwise, I don't believe they would even be included in the category of bipolar disorder. I don't think they really fit into the category of the *slowed down pole*. Their episodes of mania, if any, are minuscule. And their depressions are just different from Bipolar I depressions (*slowed down pole*).

This type of depression can go on and on without responding to any of the usual treatments. I believe that this is sometimes referred to as "treatment resistant depression" or simply TRD. My failures at treating depression were usually this type of depression. They can sleep a lot, usually at night but sometimes in the daytime. Their desire is to simply lay on the couch and do absolutely nothing. Their arms and legs may feel heavy. They hate themselves, but they just cannot get off the couch. Farmers need to feed their animals, but they just cannot get off the couch. If they have children, they will get them off to school, maybe, before lying down on the couch for the remainder of the day. Dishes stack up in the sink. The whole house is a mess. But they cannot get off the couch. Extreme passivity makes me think of this diagnosis right away even before I know that they have had tiny episodes of mania. Of course, jumping to conclusions without a thorough history is dangerous, but this marked passivity is so obvious. Getting into treatment is too much for this book. Treatment is very challenging for all psychiatrists. Of course, like all serious mental illnesses, suicide is always a possibility.

Chapter 4

MIXED MANIA

Mixed Mania was the main reason I started this book. They are frequently treated as depression with antidepressants rather than medications for mania because one of the most common presentations of mixed mania is depression.

A young girl, age 16, straight A's in school, was brought to my office by her mother. In the last couple of years, she had made six suicidal attempts and had been hospitalized four times at our local private psychiatric hospital. She had been prescribed at least four different antidepressants with no reduction in her depression. I ask her how long it took her to fall asleep at night? She replied, about four hours. I ask her if her mind was racing. Sometimes patients have a hard time answering this question, but she responded quickly in the affirmative. Racing mind and onset insomnia revealed to me that she might be having mixed mania, not depression. I gave her Depakote and Risperdal. There are many other medications for mania, but I just happened to give her these two medications. She responded quickly. The depression was gone. Her mother worked in retail. I saw her at a store about 1 1/2 years later. She was still doing very well, but she did not take these medications all the time. She was not taking the Depakote, but she took the Risperdal whenever her mind started to race and she could not fall asleep. The depression had not returned at that time. I forgot to mention that I gradually reduced and stopped her antidepressant medication. Antidepressants generally do not help mixed mania, but in the next year or two, I discovered that a few patients did better if I left them on a very low dose of antidepressants in addition to a low dose of medications for mania. Not all patients respond as perfectly as the example I gave above.

But mixed mania can also present as rage. They usually receive more appropriate treatment. There is a type of depression that presents with rage, but they do not exhibit the racing mind and insomnia that is classic for mixed mania. The people in rage do not usually receive an antidepressant. They usually receive some form of treatment (probably an antipsychotic or a mood stabilizer) that is beneficial. This form of mixed mania did not inspire me to write this book because it is usually treated adequately. But note that they do not have the extreme increase in energy typical of bipolar mania. They only have a racing mind and onset insomnia typical of mixed mania. Remember classical mania with the extreme increased energy level is dramatic, "sticks out like a sore thumb." These people tell you about their rage, but it is not obvious from behavior or speech in your office. Of course, their family members see it at home.

Very rarely, very rarely, mixed mania can present as paranoia. They feel the people on television are giving them a message, as an example. I've only seen this presentation a very few times, but they still give a history classic for mixed mania such as onset insomnia and the racing mind. My diagnostic terminology, in this case, could be in error since this presentation is so rare.

The fourth presentation of mixed mania is very dramatic. Fortunately, I have only seen it a few times beginning back in the 1960s. They have an "awful anxiety" that will not respond to the usual anxiolytics like benzodiazepines or antidepressants. At first, I think they have simple chronic anxiety easily treated. But they rapidly worsen rather than improving when I give them benzodiazepines like Valium, Klonopin, etc. Within a day or two they may voluntarily go into a psychiatric unit seeking relief if my treatment does not present results right away. It is truly an "awful anxiety" — in a class of its own. I often miss the diagnosis at first. In the hospital, they will be given medications for mania plus anxiolytics sometimes, but definitely medications for mania. Of course, like all other mixed mania, they will have the outstanding features classical for that disease — a racing mind and onset insomnia.

One time a 29-year-old woman came into my office and told me that she had mixed mania. I ask her how she knew that? She stated that she had been in our local private psychiatric hospital and her psychiatrist told her what her diagnosis was. She had had this illness since age 12. She had been given antidepressants without any help for 17 years. The diagnosis was missed for 17 years. The psychiatrist treated her successfully. Her mood disorder was under good control. But, through the years, not knowing what was wrong with her, she had turned to alcohol seeking relief. The alcoholism treatment became a great challenge. Alcoholism was more difficult to treat than mixed mania. Many people with these mood disorders, not understanding what is wrong with them, turn to alcohol or marijuana seeking relief.

Chapter 5

DEPRESSION

The syndromes of melancholia and hysteria are found in Egyptian literature as far back as 2600 BC. Hippocrates made reference to melancholia. Kraepelin described melancholia in "Lectures On Clinical Psychiatry" in 1904. Dreyfus, a physician pupil of Dr. Kraepelin, thought that agitated melancholia was an adulterated form of manic-depressive illness. Kraepelin saw it as a distinct type of depression. Controversy continued on this topic.

Is melancholia a particular type of depression? I think it is. I have described it below as one of my five types of depression. Adolph Meyer (1866-1950) advocated use of the word depression and elimination of the word melancholia. In the new *Diagnostic and Statistical Manual V*, reference is made to "melancholic symptoms," as part of the symptoms typical of depression. The small amount of historical data above comes from more than one of the "Comprehensive Textboooks of Psychiatry" authored by Freedman, Kaplan, and Saddock and later by Ruiz (Ninth Edition).

Although the new *Diagnostic and Statistical Manual V* (DSM V), authored by a committee designated by the American Psychiatric Association, describes depression in a comprehensive manner, I would like to endeavor to describe five types of depression that I have observed.

1) Normal grief or bereavement are not considered as depression in DSM V. It is true that most people suffering from loss of a loved one, usually a human being but on rare occasion a pet, do not consider their problem to be significant enough to make an appointment with a psychiatrist. But sometimes they do enter into psychotherapy with a qualified therapist to help them cope with their grief. In fact, this is not uncommon at all. Grief is not usually treated with any medication, but in very rare instances of abnormal grief of prolonged duration, it might be. Many times I am seeing a patient for another psychiatric illness and they will experience a loss and describe their grief in passing. Of course, I express my condolences, but I would tend to not dwell on their grief. Instead I would continue to focus on the original problem they came to see me about. Most of these patients cope with their grief without my help. But some people do need professional help to cope with their unusually severe grief.

2) I frequently see what I call an "Angry Type of Depression." The presenting complaint by the patient is anger, not depression. Only after a careful interrogation does it become apparent that the patient is also depressed

as well as angry. I first became aware of this type of depression while treating a 14-year-old teenager. He was always looking for a fight. If given the slightest provocation, he was eager to fight. In talking to him, he revealed that this all started at about 11 years of age when he lost his grandmother who was the only close parenting figure in his life. There was one other important symptom of depression — anhedonia. He was not receiving pleasure from anything in life. He did not exhibit any symptoms of mixed mania such as a racing mind, difficulty focusing on the task at hand, or great difficulties in falling asleep. At first, I thought this only occurred in children and teenagers. But later, many adults came to see me whose only complaint was continual inappropriate rage, or anger, or extreme irritability. The other major symptom of depression was anhedonia. They were not really enjoying anything in their life. There were not any of the other classical symptoms of depression as outlined in DSM V.

The inner critic is not so punitive in this type of depression. Consequently, in my opinion, this type of depression is a distinct entity that should not be just be lumped into the illness of depression. This diagnosis requires good communication, or repeated attempts at communication, between the psychiatrist and the patient. The diagnosis could easily be missed. Anhedonia is very important in making this diagnosis.

I had one patient, a teenage boy, who would not go to

school because of his rage. It was extremely difficult for me to make this diagnosis, or differentiate it from mixed mania. After many months, the diagnosis was finally made by the fact that he responded to a rather large dose of Lexapro (escitalopram). Lexapro is an SSRI (antidepressant) that we will talk about later. If the diagnosis were mixed mania, he would not have responded to this antidepressant. My only clue that should have helped me make the diagnosis sooner was the fact that one of his parents had a serious depression that responded to an SSRI type of antidepressant. So far, all of the patients I have seen with this type of depression responded to an SSRI type of antidepressant. As many of you know, SSRI is an abbreviation for Serotonin Specific Reuptake Inhibitor.

3) And then there is the rather classic depression as described in DSM V. The patient comes in and tells you that they are depressed. It is usually not too difficult to diagnose. But the psychiatrist should always look for any evidence of bipolar disorder. A patient may come in following a very traumatic experience and the initial diagnosis is obviously depression. But, upon further questioning, you find this patient has some past history that is definitely indicative of bipolar disorder, or at least could be indicative of bipolar disorder. Again the dx of bipolar disorder is easily missed. The most common symptoms for this type of depression, as described in DSM V, are complete lack of any pleasure in life often including sexuality,

sometimes experiencing anxiety, sometimes experiencing loss of appetite (but not always), usually awaking early in the morning after only four or five hours of sleep, often experiencing fatigue, having feelings of unrealistic guilt and worthlessness, frequently indecisive with serious loss of self-confidence in all their endeavors, and possibly impairment in social and occupational abilities. They may even have minimal to severe slowing in cognition. Also, due to their misery and feelings of worthlessness, they may strongly desire to die and have suicidal ideation. Suicidal ideation is more common than uncommon. But for some unknown reason, suicidal ideation is not always present. This is a mystery to me. In my opinion, the two symptoms that are always present are anhedonia and strong feelings of guilt and worthlessness. Multiple other symptoms of depression as described above may be present. And do not forget the inner critic. It is very punitive during these times of depression.

4) I have not seen it recently, but in years gone by I had at least a few female patients, beyond menopause, who had the classical symptoms of depression as already described above, but also they experienced an early morning anxiety or agitation that was extremely severe lasting until at least 1 p.m. daily or slightly longer. They were referred to as having involutional melancholia. The DSM V does mention agitation as a possible symptom of depression. I assume they were including this diagnosis in

their classification of depression. But this was just a different form of depression to me, and I think it is a distinct entity.

5) In years gone by, probably in the 1960s or 1970s, I saw a severely depressed man exhibiting all of the symptoms that would now be referred to as "melancholic symptoms." He had zero energy to do anything. He stared at the floor continuously. He often took deep breaths as if exhausted. During an interview, he might slowly lift his head to look at me for a brief second, one time. Speech was extremely slow and sparse. Practically no speech. He might briefly express his thoughts of extreme worthlessness. He was losing weight rapidly. His affect of depression was just much more extreme and obvious than the remainder of depressions that I have described above. If he had the energy, he would commit suicide. If an antidepressant were to partially help him, some increase in energy would make him a serious suicide risk.

I believe this is the type of patient that Dr. Max Fink would recommend for ECT. Dr. Fink was born in 1923 and spent many years in several universities in the Northeast involved in research and clinical practice. Some of his work occurred before the advent of antidepressant medications. Much of his research revolved around trying to determine the best way to administer electroconvulsive therapy (ECT), how it worked, and who would profit the most. I heard him speak one time at a large gathering of psychiatrists. I was very impressed with his commitment to research in his area of greatest interest. I believe he is still actively in practice or research at SUNY.

6) Some of these severely depressed people become psychotic. They may begin to hear voices commanding them to commit suicide. Their inner critic may become audible in the form of auditory hallucinations. These hallucinations may reason with them so that suicide sounds completely logical. The voices may continuously hammer them about their extreme multiple shortcomings as human beings. These tormented people will require some type of antipsychotic medication in addition to antidepressant medication. The hallucinations are extremely disturbing and tormenting.

The Agency for Healthcare Research And Quality Review (AHRQ), one of 12 agencies within the United States Department of Health and Human Services (DHH), reviewed the literature for treatment of depression after unsatisfactory response to SSRIs. They reviewed 46,884 citations. In their opinion, 44 studies and 27 guidelines were eligible for inclusion. Please note the number of citations they found that were not eligible for inclusion. Forty-one studies involved only adults. Three studies involved children and adolescents ages 8 through 18. Their conclusion was that "there is low strength of evidence evaluating relative differences for any monotherapy or combination therapy approach." "All but 2 of the 44 studies showed no relative difference in response and remission rates. Two studies with limited sample size using risperidone as an augmenting agent showed benefit for combined therapy." The majority of studies were not designed to evaluate superiority of switching strategies among antidepressants. Inconsistencies and lack of clarity for clinical actions were noted when comparing "Clinical Practice Guidelines." Systematic literature reviews concerning "switching strategies" among antidepressants were also found to be inconclusive.

For several years now most psychiatrists including myself have followed the American Psychiatric Association guidelines for treatment of depression including "switching strategies." Also many of us were very influenced by the Sequenced Treatment Alternatives to Relieve Depression (Star-D) study, a cooperative study among 41 study locations, with 4000 enrollees, sponsored by NIMH, and spearheaded by the University of Texas Southwestern Medical School, Department of Psychiatry, Dr. A John Rush. Even though proof of effectiveness with reference to "switching strategies" may be hard to find, I am going to personally advocate use of switching strategies until your psychiatrist finds the right antidepressant or the right combination of antidepressants to obtain a strong response or hopefully a remission with reference to your depression. Note that (AHRQ) evaluated 27 guidelines for treatment of depression. If you have been depressed for months or years without relief, get another medical opinion or change psychiatrists. I would give my own patients the same advice, "go see a different psychiatrist." Any psychiatrist who would put a patient on a certain antidepressant medication and leave them on the same medication for several years without much response, and certainly without remission, is practicing a very inferior brand of psychiatry. Change, change, change, if the first trial of an antidepressant is ineffective. And many first trials are ineffective. I have received patients who have been on one single antidepressant medication for 3-5 years with minimal if any response. That is tragic.

There are five Serotonin Specific Reuptake Inhibitors (SSRI). They were the first of the newer antidepressants following the older tricyclic antidepressants. The tricyclic antidepressants were effective, probably as effective as SSRIs, but they had more pronounced side effects. The tricylic antidepressants became available in the mid-1960s. The SSRIs became available in the late 1980s and early 1990s. The older tricyclic antidepressants are rarely used today.

SSRIs inhibit the reuptake of serotonin into special storage vesicles in the neurons causing more serotonin to be available for chemical neurotransmission in certain areas of the brain important for mood regulation. SNRIs inhibit the reuptake of serotonin and norepinephrine into their respective storage vesicles in the neurons so that more of both are available for chemical neurotransmission between neurons in areas of the brain important for mood regulation. The SSRIs first released to the public were Prozac, Paxil, and Zoloft. Later Celexa and Lexapro became available. The SNRI's that have come into common use are Effexor, Cymbalta, and Pristiq. I have used the brand names rather than the generic names.

Stimulants such as Ritalin (methylphenidate) and various forms of amphetamines (Dexedrine, Adderall, and Vyvanse) cause more norepinephrine and dopamine to be available for chemical neurotransmission. They are controlled substances because of the increase in dopamine for neurotransmission. Dopamine is responsible for the 'high" in all "feel good" substances. They are sometimes used to augment the above mentioned classical antidepressants when all else fails.

You now have all three neurotransmitters known to be effective in mood regulation. They are serotonin, norepinephrine, and dopamine. A great deal of research is now in progress to determine how some of the other major neurotransmitters may enter in to mood regulation, such as glutamate and GABA (gamma amino butyric acid). But for the past several years, three neurotransmitters manipulated for mood regulation, were serotonin, norepinephrine, and dopamine. Too much of any of these three neurotransmitters could cause hypertensive crises. That is why one must be very careful when combining antidepressant medications. These crises are called "serotonergic syndrome." It is rare, but it must always be kept in mind when prescribing more than one antidepressant medication at the same time to a single patient. Dopamine is the "feel good" neurotransmitter responsible for a "high" caused by alcohol, narcotics, marijuana, stimulants as listed above, sexual stimulation, etc., etc. Any medication responsible for additional dopamine in the brain for chemical neurotransmission could be addictive. That maybe the reason that stimulants are only added to antidepressants when other combinations have all failed.

Note that the brain reacts to additional dopamine by decreasing the number of dopamine receptors. Consequently, more and more of the drug that caused the pleasure must be taken to continue that effect. When the drug is stopped, a terrible depression follows due to the reduction in dopamine receptors in the brain. That is why cocaine users need more and more of that drug to obtain the "high" they obtained with their first use. Their brain reacts to cocaine (causing more dopamine) by decreasing the number of dopamine receptors, thus defeating the cocaine. So they need more and more cocaine, but if they cease to use it, they will have a severe depression — due to less dopamine receptors.

Dopamine receptors are needed for almost any sort of pleasure. As I understand it, the "depression from hell" is even worse following cessation of use of narcotics.

Unfortunately some people fight their depression by turning to these drugs of addiction when they are extremely depressed.

Sometimes mood stabilizers may be added to an SSRI or SNRI, such as lithium or Lamictal (lamotrigine) to augment the classical antidepressants. These drugs are more commonly used for the treatment of bipolar disorders. Sometimes a form of thyroid hormone (T3) triiodothyronine is added to augment the more classical antidepressants. I did see some research showing that T3 is considerably more effective than lithium as an augmenting agent, but it is rarely used in clinical practice.

There are two other classical antidepressants used to augment SSRIs and SNRIs, namely mirtazapine and bupropion. Five research projects showed that mirtazapine causes a more rapid response than SSRIs or SNRIs, but they were all funded by the manufacturers of mirtazapine. But some psychiatrists would use mirtazapine as their first trial against the depression.

I will try to give you my simplified approach to a "switching strategy" which is very much influenced by the APA guidelines and the STAR-D study. This is my "bottom line" for the treatment of depression. Most psychiatrists including myself would start with a SSRI. In the past, many of us would have tried a second SSRI before starting an SNRI, but more recent research has shown that Effexor (venlafaxine), an SNRI, is slightly more likely than any SSRI to cause a response if tried first. So now I would first try an SSRI and then try an SNRI before starting any augmentation with Remeron (mirtazapine) or Wellbutrin (bupropion).

Each medication must be given four to eight weeks to calculate the response, if any. Remission is rarely obtained on the first trial. The dose of each medication must be increased gradually. The patient must be observed over time for response. If no response occurs after a certain period of time, switching or augmentation is a must. All psychiatrists know these dosages and time needed to evaluate for response. Most readers would be overwhelmed with minutia if I attempted to elaborate on dosages. So I have elected not to discuss dosages which are all available online or from your pharmacist. Also the side effects are quickly available from multiple other sources. Very frequently, a simple change from an SSRI to an SNRI, or vice versa, may be all that is needed to obtain a response. Of course, with time or augmentation, we hope that a response will lead to remission. If there is no response, it is almost impossible that a remission could occur from that medication given a longer period of time.

Sometimes in a hospital setting, due to pressure from managed-care, a change from one antidepressant to another must be made rather quickly looking for a response. If we see a response from an antidepressant, we are hoping that further outpatient care will lead to a remission in the depression. Sometimes a psychiatrist will think that he observes a response, but after one or two months of observation, he realizes he was wrong.

I lost a patient to suicide once in the 1970s. He responded to amitriptyline, I thought, but after about five weeks I realized that he was not continuing to improve. I was going to change to desipramine at his 10:30 a.m. appointment on a Wednesday morning. But very unfortunately, he shot himself in the head that morning before the appointment.

In those days, I used amitriptyline, which caused a higher proportion of the neurotransmitter serotonin, and then switched to desipramine, which caused a higher proportion of norepinephrine. Currently we are doing somewhat the same thing, but using newer drugs which have less side effects. These older drugs were called tricyclic antidepressants as I mentioned earlier.

Let me back up for a moment and summarize the available antidepressants that are predominantly in use today. The SSRIs are Prozac, Paxil, Zoloft, Celexa, and Lexapro. The SNRIs are Effexor, Cymbalta, and Pristiq. I have given you the brand names only. First, switching occurs usually between groups. If an SSRI is ineffective, perhaps an SNRI will be effective. Two other antidepressants usually used for augmentation are Remeron and Wellbutrin. Other substances used for augmentation, if all else fails, are lithium, Lamictal, Cytomel, Ritalin, and some form of amphetamine such as Dexedrine, Adderall, or Vyvanse. If the patient is depressed with psychotic features, hearing voices, etc. an antipsychotic medication of some sort becomes essential to treat the psychosis. Some trial and error may be needed here, but I will discuss antipsychotic medications in another chapter.

If the patient has severe insomnia, either before falling asleep or awaking too early, some medication for insomnia may be necessary to obtain a good remission. In fact, without sleep, remission from depression may be impossible. Most people need seven to eight hours per night for optimum physical and mental health. Many people are forced to get by with less because of sleep disturbances by their family members, or due to demands from their work. They can tolerate this somewhat better in their younger years, but as they age, their bodies will show multiple evidences of lack of proper sleep. Just the opposite of bipolar mania, most depressed patients will be able to fall asleep, but they will awaken early in the morning having gotten only five, maybe six, hours of sleep. A later chapter on insomnia points out that they may need a small amount of sleep medication early in the morning when they awake. Some authorities would worry about some sedation while driving to work the next morning. Each patient is different and will require different treatments for insomnia.

Some people will need treatment of anxiety. There is practically no good research that shows any particular antidepressant treats both depression and anxiety effectively at the same time. (I hope I am quoting AHRQ accurately). There was one or two studies that showed that Effexor might treat anxiety in addition to depression. Benzodiazepines are controversial, as I have discussed in a different chapter, but low dosages may be needed in addition to antidepressant medications for treatment of anxiety.

The angry type depression, in my own limited number of patients, will usually respond to an SSRI. The slowed down bipolar type depression may not respond to any antidepressant alone. But, I usually have more luck with an SNRI for this bipolar type depression. My experience is mostly with Effexor. But SNRI's are not always the antidepressant of choice for the slowed down bipolar depression. Sometimes my patient tells me that they have responded best to an SSRI in the past.

In taking a history concerning their depression, it is obvious that the psychiatrist should ask about their previous experiences with antidepressants. This may help the psychiatrist find the right antidepressant sooner with fewer trials.

There were 16 studies to find out if antidepressants increased suicidal ideation in children under 18 years of age. Five of the 16 studies said yes. Eleven of the 16 studies said no. But, the usual practice is to tell every young person and their parents that starting an antidepressant could worsen suicidal ideation. The information above about the studies concerning antidepressants causing increased suicidal ideation in the young is hopefully an accurate quote from AHRQ. If the young person had mixed mania, often erroneously diagnosed as depression, the antidepressant might make him or her more agitated and possibly more suicidal. The latest advice for treating very young depressed patients is to start with a very low-dose and proceed cautiously.

There is good research to support long-term use of the effective combination of antidepressants and augmenting agents to prevent relapse, if the depression occurs more than one time. Every patient with first time depression should continue the successful treatment for at least one year, maybe longer, but they deserve a period of time without antidepressants to see what happens. Some people will need antidepressant medication treatment indefinitely to prevent multiple relapses throughout their life. Just like diabetes, most people need continued treatment after it starts. This is true for many physical ailments. This may be even more important for the treatment of children. Multiple serious episodes of depression in children is likely to lead to suicidal attempts because children are more impulsive than adults.

A lot of money and time is being poured into research concerning the genetics of the major mental illnesses. In the future, diagnoses of mental illness will be based on genetics, neurochemistry, and other hard evidence of the diagnosis. But currently, we are still making diagnoses based on our clinical experience and what the patient tells us. My limited knowledge of the genetics of depression is that some people have the genetic makeup to be more or less immune to depression, unless the stressors that cause depression are severe. Other people are just average. They could get depressed depending on the stressors they encounter during their lifetime. Some people, by genetics, are almost doomed to be depressed unless they are just very lucky. There is obviously considerable knowledge of the genetics of depression that I am not including in this book. But the diagnosis at this time is still based on clinical evaluation by the psychiatrist or family physician.

The most common adverse events due to antidepressant medication are diarrhea, dizziness, dry mouth, fatigue, sexual dysfunction, headaches, nausea, sweating, tremor, and weight gain. The severity and duration of the side effects are important in determining which antidepressants the patient can tolerate. These are distressing side effects, but they leave no permanent damage when the antidepressant is discontinued. Also SSRIs diminish blood clotting to some extent. This could be important if they are taken with anticoagulants, aspirin products, etc.

A discussion of the safety of taking antidepressants during pregnancy is beyond the scope of this book.

Chapter 6

ADDRESSING THE PREJUDICE AGAINST BENZODIAZEPINES

Today, I feel there is a prejudice in the vast majority of the medical community, and especially the mental health community, against benzodiazepines. This extends to registered nurses, social workers, psychologists, and psychiatrists. They believe benzodiazepines are highly addictive. They believe that they are deadly in overdosage. They are absolutely certain in their prejudice against benzodiazepines. I call this a prejudice because these beliefs are not supported by research or facts. As a prescriber of benzodiazepines, I frequently feel the disapproval of my fellow healthcare workers.

These beliefs originated sometime in the 1980s and are perpetuated by almost all current teachers in psychiatry from generation to generation. Since everyone is so certain of their knowledge about benzodiazepines, they simply "parrot" their beliefs among each other. Parrots are birds who just repeat what other people say. Although it does not take much courage to speak up in favor of benzodiazepines, it is rarely done. When I try to talk to my younger colleagues about this prejudice, they are absolutely certain that I am in error. They have avoided benzodiazepines. They really do not have much experience with them. But, sometimes I am gratified to find younger psychiatrists who think as I do about benzodiazepines. I wish I could associate with these bright young psychiatrists more often. I do not detect this prejudice in older psychiatrists who were trained before 1985.

People who need this medication for treatment of their severe, miserable, generalized anxiety disorders are often looked upon as "drug seeking." Or maybe they seek it for treatment of very frightening panic attacks. Possibly they are seeking it for treatment of a very miserable "mixed mania" with a racing mind and sometimes severe anxiety, and sometimes paranoia.

Benzodiazepines alone will not successfully treat "mixed mania," but they can be of great value. They will usually need mood stabilizers, antipsychotics, etc. Unfortunately these people do not understand this. The benzodiazepine will help, but not enough, and they will want to take larger and larger dosages leading to fairly serious physical dependence, which can occur with almost any sedative medication. These same people, in desperation, not really understanding what is wrong with them, will also use alcohol or marijuana trying to slow their racing mind. Forever after they will be looked upon as "addicts." If I were to give one of them a benzodiazepine, my colleagues will say that I am giving a benzodiazepine to an addict. This has been used against me in hospital politics on more than one occasion.

I hypothesize that much of the prejudice against benzodiazepines originates with the professionals who treat primarily substance abuse disorders. They are constantly "banging the drum" as to how addictive benzodiazepines are. Although they are controlled substances, I do not feel that they belong in the same class of addictive drugs as narcotics, alcohol, marijuana, cocaine, methamphetamine, etc. I say that because benzodiazepines do not cause a "high" like these other controlled substances do. Most patients use benzodiazepines, sometimes for 30 or 40 years, without ever escalating the dose, and they are still effective in controlling their generalized anxiety disorder, panic disorder, or social phobia. The leaders in the field of psychiatry are constantly advising treating these disorders with newer antidepressant medications called SSRIs or SNRIs. Cochran Collaboration, a worldwide organization that evaluates the quality of research, finds that only one in five patients with these disorders will respond to these antidepressant medications. So perhaps only 20 or 30 percent of people with these anxiety disorders will respond to these antidepressants. This is why so many patients come to me who have been taking antidepressants for two to five years with practically no relief of their anxiety disorders.

In blissful ignorance, I first used Valium (diazepam) about 1964. I gave it for 15 years with no side effects to speak of and no known addictions. The practice was of limited size in a relatively affluent area of the West Coast. Most of these people were working in the aerospace industry at that time attempting to put a man on the moon. Often it was family members I was treating. Valium was extremely beneficial, almost 100 percent, for treatment of generalized anxiety disorders, panic attacks, and a very limited number of patients with social phobias.

Many of the best psychopharmacologists in the United States are aware that antidepressants are not that effective in the treatment of generalized anxiety disorders, panic attacks, and social phobias. But, in my opinion, due to the severe prejudice against benzodiazepines, all they will say in their writings on this topic is that benzodiazepines can be given initially for rapid relief until the antidepressant takes effect, or that benzodiazepines can be added to supplement the antidepressant. But they do not give the benzodiazepine much credit for alleviating their miseries. The prejudice is powerful. Below, I will quote a well-respected textbook in the late 1990s using excellent research which extended for longer than 20 years showing that most patients use benzodiazepines for many years for control of their chronic anxiety issues with no escalation of the dose.

"Textbook Of Psychopharmacology," published by

the American Psychiatric Press in 1994 and again in 1998. Authors were Schatzberg and Nemeroff. I will be quoting from the first edition in 1994.

> *As a class, benzodiazepines have remarkably few side effects, the principal one being sedation. Patients reported feeling sedated, drowsy, and slowed down, and may fall asleep during daytime activities, or have ataxia or slurred speech. (Linnoila 1983). In laboratory settings, slowed psychomotor performance has been observed (Hindmarch et al. 1981). Amnesia (anterograde) also occurs with intravenous administration, an effective use widely in anesthesia induction (King 1992). But it has also been reported with oral dosing, especially with hypnotic triazolam (Greenblatt et al. 1991). Amnesia is also present in a less dramatic fashion in routine use, some patients reporting relatively minor difficulties in learning new material (Barbee 1993; Ghoneim and Merwalt 1990; Greenboatt 1991; Hindmarch et al. 1991; King 1992; Linnoila et al. 1983; Miller et al. 1998; Roth et al. 1984; Schader et al. 1986). However, the side effects are generally transient and disappear quickly (usually within days) as tolerance to these effects develops (Miller et al. 1988).*
>
> *The controversy surrounding benzodiazepine administration and potential abuse or addiction in routine patient use is generally not supported by*

the available scientific evidence. (See Schader and Greenblatt 1993 for an excellent review of this complex area). In a large community study of long-term alprazolam users, Romach and colleagues (1992) found that dosage did not escalate over prolonged use and that most patients use the benzodiazepines as prescribed. In fact, if deviations occurred, it was generally that a patient took less than the prescribed dose.

Evidence regarding the use of benzodiazepines during pregnancy is inconclusive. For this reason it is prudent to postpone pregnancy until benzodiazepine treatment has been discontinued. In addition, because benzodiazepines are excreted through the breastmilk and place the child at risk for lethargy and inadequate temperature regulation, nursing mothers should also be cautioned against the use of benzodiazepines (Bernstein 1988)."

Discontinuation

For the sake of thoroughness, a statement regarding discontinuation of benzodiazepines is in order. (See Ballenger et al. 1993; Schader and Greenblatt 1993.) Numerous groups, including some medical professionals, have perpetuated the idea that if used in the long term, patients become "addicted" to the benzodiazepines, resulting in an extreme withdrawal syndrome when the medication is discontinued. Actually, what occurs with benzodiazepines is similar to the effects of other medications used for long-term treatment of a medical and/or psychiatric condition, and that can be compared to what happens when a patient's cardiovascular medicine (e.g. propranolol, methyldopa) is suddenly discontinued (Garbus et al. 1979). In essence, the body goes through an adaptation process to the drug, and if medication is discontinued too abruptly, the patient can experience withdrawal symptoms. In the case of a patient treated for anxiety conditions, the patient may experience a transient recurrence of anxiety symptoms, often at levels more intense than those experienced before treatment. This is called rebound. Patients can also experience a return of symptoms that were present before treatment (relapse). However, if dosage is adjusted and a gradually titrated downward, and if the patients and their families are educated about what to expect during the discontinuation process, most patients can manage the transit withdrawal symptoms without much difficulty. (See Ballenger et al. 1993 and Schader and Greenblatt 1993 for review.)

Yes, I do pick the research that agrees with my clinical experience. Or, I wait until better research comes along. (Please detect an element of humor here.) Actually, there may be a few people who have terrible withdrawals from benzodiazepines. There is some smoke to support this, and where there is smoke, there is often some fire. There is a website called "benzobuddies" which describes the terrible experiences some people are going through in discontinuing benzodiazepines. I don't know what to think about this. Perhaps you should go to that website and come to your own conclusions. But I know that the vast majority of people do not have these types of "weird experiences" discontinuing benzodiazepines. It is not unusual for a patient to tell me, several months later, that they spontaneously discontinued a benzodiazepine without my knowledge. They speak of it casually as if it was a nonevent. If I should question them about withdrawal, they talk and act as if it was a nonevent.

Contradictory research is more common than uncommon. The topic of contradictory research could easily be a chapter or a book in its own right. When you see research quoted in one of the major newspapers in our country, take it with a grain of salt. New and sensational findings make good press. People read it. It is entertaining. But the conclusions may not be true.

As clinicians, we often know something before the research is written to support our knowledge. Psychiatrists were using Depakote (valproic acid) for the treatment of bipolar disorder several years before the FDA approved it for that use. As many of you know, it was originally used to control seizures. Several psychiatrists, including myself, were aware that Abilify (aripiprazole) would augment antidepressants before the FDA approved it for that use. Now, most of my patients have seen the advertisements on television.

At a large national psychopharmacology conference in February 2014, I was told that there is no research to support the use of Lamictal (lamotrigine) as a mood stabilizer for bipolar mania. In fact, four research projects were negative for beneficial results in controlling mania. But I see patients who seem to be benefiting greatly from the use of lamotrigine for control of mania. And other psychiatrists have told me of their good experiences using lamotrgine as a mood stabilizer.

Hopefully you can understand why clinicians do value their clinical experience as well as research findings. On any given topic, the Cochrane Collaboration may find, out of several thousand bits of research, only 40 to 80 worthy of inclusion in their studies. I will ignore any single research study that obviously goes against my clinical experience and common sense knowledge. But a group like NIDA (National Institute For Drug Abuse) may use that same piece of research to support their opinion concerning benzodiazepines or the legalization of marijuana, etc. I am probably guilty of the same thing. I would probably believe research that supports my viewpoints garnered from clinical experience.

National organizations like NIDA are not infallible. But NIDA supported research and professional education have been very valuable to my understanding of substance abuse and addiction problems. I simply said they are not infallible.

This prejudice against benzodiazepines is well known among patients, and perhaps even among the general public. I have had people from the community, who hardly knew me, asking me to try to convince the other psychiatrists in this area as to the value of benzodiazepines for treating emotional illness. One man was on total disability due to severe and frequent panic attacks. He was taking Xanax (alprazolam) 1 mg four times per day. He was a collector of antiques, and I met him because my wife is also interested in collectibles. When I first moved to Shreveport, Louisiana in 1991, practicing anesthesia, he was trying to convince me to tell the psychiatrists in this area how valuable benzodiazepines are for the treatment of panic attacks. Many psychiatrists will not prescribe them simply to protect themselves, not necessarily in the best interest of their patients. There is a market on the street for benzodiazepines. Perhaps they are genuinely fearful of being duped. Others fully buy into the prejudice against them for whatever reason.

Unfortunately, certain experiences will strengthen the prejudice against benzodiazepines dramatically. A certain type of personality, often referred to in medical circles as an "addictive personality," will use any mind altering substance they can obtain. They will sniff glue. They will use LSD, mescaline, rare plants found only in certain mountains of Mexico, etc., etc. To some extent, benzodiazepines are mind altering. A very rare patient may even find them to cause a "high." This does not mean that they will use them inappropriately. But people with an "addictive personality" will use them inappropriately. Some people on the streets, not addictive personalities, have emotional problems that are relieved by benzodiazepines. The prejudice against benzodiazepines may have made it difficult for them to obtain them in a legal manner. These people may obtain benzodiazepines illegally, even though they are not "addicts."

When emotionally ill people use benzodiazepines (along with multiple other medications) for a suicide attempt, this leaves an indelible impression on the minds of many mental health workers. It is almost a knee-jerk reaction among mental health professionals these days to blame the benzodiazepine for a suicide attempt, the traffic accident, a fall in the hallway, etc., even though the benzodiazepine may not be at all to blame. Mental health professionals will often mention first in their progress notes that the patient was taking a benzodiazepine when these accidents occurred. The prescriber, often me, is thus immediately blamed for whatever has happened. This is because prescribers of benzodiazepines are looked down upon by many other mental health professionals, especially young people educated since 1985. Some are physicians, but some are not physicians. They believe what they have been taught. If they work in substance abuse, the condemnation will be even more severe.

Emotionally disturbed people make suicide attempts. This makes a bad impression on EMT professionals rushing the patient to the emergency room. The benzodiazepine did not cause the overdosage. The misery of the emotional illness caused the overdosage. Many other medications may also have been taken, and some of them cause cardiac dysrhythmias more deadly than simple sedation. Benzodiazepines in overdosage could cause the patient to sleep in their apartment for several days without dying. Benzodiazepines do not usually depress respirations to the point of death unless they are mixed with other sedative medications such as alcohol, narcotics, etc. When they are, they do contribute to death. But if the patient reaches the emergency room, the ER doctor can reverse the effects of benzodiazepines very effectively to prevent death.

Many psychiatrists in private practice, including myself, will have a contract which the patient must sign in order to obtain benzodiazepines, if needed. If they request refills ahead of time, if they are obtaining them from another physician, if any evidence arises that they are not taking them as prescribed, the doctor-patient relationship can be terminated or the benzodiazepine can be discontinued. Unfortunately, I have had to do this from time to time. I cannot afford to continue to prescribe this controlled substance to that individual. There is a website in many states, sponsored by a state agency, where the physician can find out if this patient is obtaining a controlled substance from more than one physician.

I think every medical professional should keep in mind that benzodiazepines have a very, very low incidence of side effects in comparison to most other medications. Several medications in common use can cause liver failure. Some medications could adversely affect kidneys, or cognition, or hearing. Some medications can cause tendon ruptures, neuropathies, etc. Some psychiatric medications may cause side effects resembling parkinsonism, or serious weight gain, or diabetes. Benzodiazepines are not guilty of any of these serious side effects. Maybe this is an appropriate time to mention that one benzodiazepine, Valium, may have unexpected sedative effects because about one in 25 patients do not have the necessary liver enzymes to metabolize Valium. This is very rare. I've only seen it one time in 40 years. But people starting Valium, for the first pill should only bite off a corner of it and see that they are not overly sedated. Then they can take the whole pill.

In spite of their "terrible reputation" they are the most frequently prescribed psychotropic medications in the United States and around the world. I have read the evaluation of benzodiazepines by the World Health Organization. They initiated an investigation of the appropriate use of benzodiazepines and the addiction potential in 1992. They published it in 1996. They made it very clear, as best I can understand, that no one is allowed to copy their evaluation or use it in a book like this one. I believe they said in a nutshell, "don't throw the baby out with the bathwater."

In the next few pages, I will very superficially mention the most common side effects I have seen with each of the benzodiazepines used most frequently by the medical profession today. Valium—remember that some people cannot metabolize it. I've seen it once in 40 years. But, have the patient bite off a corner of the tablet and check for sedation before giving the whole tablet.

I prefer Valium to Klonopin. A very few patients prefer Klonopin. The stigma of benzodiazepines is least with Klonopin. Rarely a patient will develop ataxia (loss of coordination in the legs) due to Klonopin. The problem disappears as soon as the medication is stopped.

Ativan (lorazepam) is a miracle worker IV in the hospital. It can be very beneficial for anxiety when given orally on an outpatient basis. But, it is a wonderful amnestic for anesthesiology. Sometimes this is a problem when given orally on an outpatient basis. I have one outstanding case in my mind where a man lost a good paying job because of confusion while working. He never could find another job of that desirability again, although the Ativan was discontinued by myself. He lost his wife. The last time I saw him he was going with his second wife to live with her parents in a small town in Arkansas. He also had bipolar disorder.

Xanax (alprazolam) is the "panic buster." It is also beneficial for insomnia because it is of short duration, about four hours. The effects can be completely gone in the morning while the patient is driving to work. This one has the worst reputation as a benzodiazepine because it is highly preferred by many patients. Rapid onset. Could easily become dependent if trying to treat bipolar mania with it. This latter statement is true of all of the benzodiazepines. Usually given in the emergency room for panic attacks along with a paper bag to breathe into. People tend to hyperventilate during a panic attack. The paper bag is given to retain carbon dioxide and restore their acid-base balance. Some people who know say that a panic attack is worse than a heart attack. I regret that I have used it so seldom because of the stigma.

I can honestly say that none of my patients taking a benzodiazepine have had a motor vehicle accident. They adapt to the mildly sedative properties very quickly. But, I would still warn any patient to be very careful when starting a new medication until they know the possible side effects for them. There are a few very sedative benzodiazepines not mentioned above and almost never given for panic or anxiety. One of them is used for seizure control.

Last I will tell you a few stories to dramatize the effectiveness of benzodiazepines for the treatment of certain illnesses I have already mentioned several times.

An executive from a small city came to see me for treatment of a severe generalized miserable anxiety disorder. He was wearing a diaper. Another psychiatrist, trying to avoid benzodiazepines, had given him an antipsychotic medication (Risperdal), an antidepressant, and a third medication I cannot remember. He was still in misery. I discontinued all three medications and simply gave him Valium 5 mg three times per day. He threw his diaper away. End of problem.

A member of my family was having severe panic attacks about 4 p.m. daily. She was in her 80s. Everyone has heard about sundowners syndrome, but this had nothing to do with sundowners syndrome. I sent her to two of the brightest psychiatrists in this area. They gave her several different types of medications trying to stop these panic attacks without using a benzodiazepine. Nothing helped. She felt as if they were in her stomach; she groaned as if they were unbearable; she could hardly stand it. She went back to her small hometown in Kansas.

Her family physician gave her Xanax four times per day. End of problem.

In 1996 I treated a very physically fit and athletic middle-aged male for panic attacks which were of recent onset. We searched, but we could not find any precipitating factor. I gave him Valium of long duration to prevent panic attacks. I also gave him a few Xanax to stop panic attacks when they occurred in spite of the Valium. I left that practice to take employment in another city. Our doctor-patient relationship was terminated. About 15 years later he brought a member of his family to see me. He did not remember my name, but after talking a few minutes, we recognized each other. He had forgotten that he ever had panic attacks. But I remembered him and that he did have panic attacks. Apparently he took the benzodiazepines for a short period of time. The panic attacks subsided and he never used the benzodiazepines again. End of problem.

I mentioned earlier that benzodiazepines are now being given for anxiety to patients with schizophrenia, schizoaffective disorder, bipolar mania, etc. Patients are usually treated with antipsychotic medications to hopefully stop or reduce auditory hallucinations, thought disorders of which there are several, etc. One patient told me that these antipsychotic medications helped him to "attend to business." Often people with schizophrenia have so much going on in their mind that they cannot attend to reality, such as bathing, paying their bills, eating properly, etc., but they do suffer from depression and anxiety also. Consequently, they can often profit from treatment with either antidepressants or benzodiazepines.

The most dramatic example of this that I can give you is that of a patient in a wheelchair in a state of psychosis hearing voices, etc. I treated her with an antipsychotic medication which fortunately helped with her auditory hallucinations and thought disorder. She was in a psychiatric unit about 1995. Theoretically, as best we could tell, she was ready for discharge to her home and further treatment on an outpatient basis. The nursing staff at the hospital knew her from previous admissions. They kept telling me that she could walk. She told me that she was paralyzed, and she never got out of her wheelchair. I guessed that this might be a conversion reaction which was either relieving anxiety or depression, I wasn't sure which. Conversion reactions manifest as physical disabilities such as loss of sensation in an extremity, loss of the ability to move an extremity, blindness, etc. These physical disabilities of emotional etiology somehow relieve the emotional discomfort of anxiety or depression. I decided to give her a benzodiazepine in case she was experiencing anxiety. After starting the benzodiazepine, she got out of the wheelchair and walked. End of story.

In February 2014, after writing the above chapter, I attended the 19th Annual Psychopharmacology Update in

Las Vegas sponsored by the Nevada Psychiatric Association. This is a well-attended annual conference. I believe there were approximately 1300 psychiatrists, psychologists, and nurse practitioners in attendance. Dr. Murray B Stein, MD, MPH, Professor of Psychiatry and Family and Preventive Medicine, University of California in San Diego delivered a lecture entitled "Attacking Anxiety Disorders." He covered most of the pertinent research discussing all the medications investigated for the treatment of anxiety disorders. He pointed out that better than 20 percent of the population of the United States experiences an anxiety disorder at some time during their lives. After covering the research findings, especially concerning antidepressants, but also other medications, he asked how many of the mental health workers in the audience used benzodiazepines. A young psychiatrist, who seemed very bright and enthusiastic, sitting next to me, quickly raised his hand. I quickly raised my hand. I looked over the audience of 1300 people as rapidly as I could. I think that less than 10 percent of the audience raised their hand. After asking the question, Dr. Stein stated that he does use benzodiazepines. He did not say how often or under what circumstances. He did not encourage the use of benzodiazepines; he simply stated that he does use them. I was very happy and encouraged to hear this. No other lecturer, during the remainder of the 32 hours I was listening, admitted to using benzodiazepines. The prejudice is powerful!

This is the third time I have written this book. This has been a long chapter, but I must add two bits of information that I have acquired since the last publishing. My last practice was with substance abusers. They tell me that they do not get a "high" out of benzodiazepines. But, I have had at least two patients, maybe more, who tried to take all of the medication I had given them for a month attempting to get a "high." They became sedated and uncoordinated. But they did not obtain a "high." Fortunately, each time, a close relative informed me of what they had done. Apparently, they were not aware that benzodiazepines do not cause a high. This frightened me, and I discontinued benzodiazepines immediately. But, people with substance abuse problems told me that Valium can enhance the effects of alcohol. Sometimes they take Valium for this reason. One cocaine user told me that he uses Valium to take the edge off of a cocaine "high." So, I cannot say that substance abusers do not use benzodiazepines. But, I have given them to hundreds of patients who took them exactly as prescribed never increasing the dose for as long as 10 or 15 years. Consequently, I think they should be used for the treatment of emotional miseries when appropriate. They should not be avoided completely as if they were deadly or addictive medications. They do not deserve the reputation they have among many younger psychiatrists.

The DEA, medical boards, etc. feel that giving benzodiazepines along with buprenorphine, a certain type of narcotic, usually referred to by the brand names of Subutex or Suboxone etc. used to help substance abusers stop using heroin, methamphetamines, etc is strongly contraindicated. It is true that the combination is definitely more lethal in overdosage than buprenorphine alone. But an overdosage of that magnitude would be a suicidal attempt. It would not be an accident. The benzodiazepine did not cause the suicidal attempt. The combination does offer an easy way out of life. Perhaps they would be afraid to use a gun or to hang themselves. But if they were really determined to commit suicide, they could find other ways to do it. There is some research from one of the Scandinavian countries who have extensive electronic health records and nationalized health insurance that people taking the combination are slightly less inclined to commit suicide than those taking only buprenorphine. Perhaps the benzodiazepine was being used to treat an emotional misery diminishing the likelihood of a suicide attempt. I have only seen one such study from Scandinavia. This was primarily a statistical study from the electronic health records of several million people.

There have been 14 studies, to my knowledge, to decide if benzodiazepines might increase the likelihood of developing dementia as we age. Eight said definitely not. Six said maybe. Sometimes the authors did not distinguish between association and causality. An aging individual who is developing dementia might experience considerable anxiety or serious insomnia. A benzodiaze-pine might be prescribed. This would be a case of associa-tion, but not causality. To my knowledge, current research shows that benzodiazepines do not increase the likelihood of developing dementia.

It is interesting that so many research studies were done concerning benzodiazepines and dementia. To my thinking this simply illustrates the prejudice against ben-zodiazepines. What about the multiple other medica-tions we prescribe in psychiatry such as antidepressants and antipsychotics, etc. sometimes for 10 years or longer? In comparison, how many research studies have been done concerning these medications as possible causes of dementia?

Chapter 7

GENERALIZED ANXIETY DISORDER AND PANIC ATTACKS

The Diagnostic and Statistical Manual V (DSM V) puts some emphasis on the origin of the anxiety. In my experience, the anxiety starts rather suddenly with no obvious cause whatsoever. The typical onset was often between 30 and 45 years of age. Most authorities believe that this is much more common in women than men, but I had at least an equal number of men and women patients suffering from this problem. Generalized Anxiety Disorder (GAD) was not associated with any real threat such as serious medical illnesses, financial problems, etc. If there was an obvious source of anxiety, I would not have classified it as an emotional illness. It was a terrible, miserable anxiety totally unrelated to reality. Sometimes it seemed to have a hereditary basis. Sometimes the patient's mother would have a similar type of illness. If it were related to past painful or frightening experience, it would be classified as Post Traumatic Stress Disorder, not GAD. If it occurred early in the onset of mixed mania, it would be classified as bipolar disorder, mixed mania. If it occurred relative to social appearance or performance, it would be classified as social phobia. If it was a child fearful of leaving the parent to attend school, it would be classified as Separation Anxiety. I will avoid discussion of social phobias, separation anxiety, and PTSD at this time. GAD and panic attacks will be the focus of the remainder of this chapter.

This Generalized Anxiety Disorder could attach momentarily to work performance, physical well-being, stability of their marriage, school performance in higher education, etc. But these were temporary attachments. They were brief and fleeting. Usually these feelings of anxiety are experienced in the abdomen and centered around a feeling of "impending doom." My experience was that they lasted a few years to 40 years. Some experts in the field of psychiatry believe that this severe generalized anxiety disorder is a major cause of suicide. But everyone agrees that bipolar depression, of one type or another, is the most frequent cause of suicide.

Another type of anxiety I saw came with prolonged periods of stress. One patient was on call 24 hours a day, 7 days a week, for a large manufacturing concern for many years. He would wake up early in the morning with nausea and vomiting. His appetite was almost gone. He was losing weight. He could obtain some relief with low-dose Xanax on awakening. After a month or so, he had to stop working. He was on sick leave for approximately six months. With rest, this condition subsided. His appetite returned; his self-confidence returned; he did not need Xanax any longer. He returned to work, but his new position was less stressful for him. This is an example of another type of anxiety, but it is different from generalized anxiety disorder. Rarely GAD did occur following periods of unusual stress, but usually the cause was a total mystery. And if GAD did occur following periods of unusual stress, the illness had a life of its own sometimes lasting for years after the stress ceased.

I sometimes attempted to help the patient realize that he had powerful feelings of guilt which would explain his feelings of impending doom. This was purely theoretical on my part in my attempts to understand where his feelings of impending doom were coming from. These attempts on my part were futile. He might diminish the anxiety by staying extremely busy. But it is hard to stay extremely busy all of the time. Perhaps some form of meditation might have helped? But these feelings of impending doom were very powerful.

A benzodiazepine will give almost immediate relief to these patients suffering these miseries. But due to the prejudice against benzodiazepines, all psychiatrists are taught to treat GAD with SSRIs (Prozac, Paxil, Zoloft, Celexa, Lexapro). Some research I have found indicates that Effexor (venlafaxine), an SNRI, is probably more effective than SSRIs for treatment of GAD, but this may vary from patient to patient. I am constantly receiving new patients with GAD who have been treated with Prozac, Paxil, Zoloft, Celexa, and Lexapro for months at a time with no relief from their miseries. This wasted time could add up to a few years of questionable "treatment."

The Cochrane Collaboration is a huge organization employing thousands of people to evaluate the quality of any research with reference to almost any topic in the medical field, not confined solely to mental health issues at all. For an example, they also evaluate the research with reference to any antibiotic as to its effectiveness against certain organisms. The origin of their funding does not influence the outcome of their findings. They might examine 3,000 or 4,000 citations on a topic, and find 80 studies that they feel they can base their findings on, just as an example.

They examined the research with reference to the effectiveness of SSRIs in the treatment of generalized anxiety disorder. They found that they can be effective, but the number needed to treat (NNT) was five for every one definite response in comparison to placebo. To me that means only 20 percent of patients, or at best 30 percent, will respond to antidepressants. This would explain why I have seen so many patients who have not responded to an SSRI. But remember, every psychiatric resident in the United States is taught to always use antidepressants to treat generalized anxiety disorder. This needs to change. The prejudice against benzodiazepines needs to be addressed. After several years of suffering, I would give them a benzodiazepine and they would be "eternally grateful." They definitely did not want to see any other psychiatrist in whatever organization I was working with. The concerns that any physician should address before prescribing a benzodiazepine is summarized in my chapter "Addressing The Prejudice Against Benzodiazepines." The most commonly used benzodiazepines for the treatment of GAD are Valium, Klonopin, Ativan, and Xanax.

Panic disorder also comes out of nowhere, and then secondarily may cause generalized anxiety with reference to the very frightening panic attacks. I have explored the circumstances and emotions of many patients at length trying to find the origin of their panic attacks. I have never been successful in doing this. Occasionally, I can see something in their circumstances that could cause anxiety. But often, I cannot find any cause whatsoever. One time, after about four years of therapy, a very intelligent man revealed something to me that could have been causing anxiety or panic attacks. He withheld that information from me for at least four years. But usually the patient and I cannot find the cause or causes.

A panic attack is accompanied by heart palpitations, a frightening feeling of not being able to breathe, chest pain, dizzy feelings, numbness around the mouth and fingers, a powerful feeling that they are losing their mind or "going crazy." One of my patients in Los Angeles talked about "running amok" which is an old Pacific islands term. In Los Angeles, this was very prone to happen in a car on the freeways surrounded by five lanes of traffic going at least 70 mph. Where do you run? What can you do? They can have a terrible feeling of being trapped. They often occur in other situations where the patient does not feel in control, such as on an elevator. They are physically and mentally painful. They are a terrible feeling. The patient always develops a severe anxiety about the recurrence of these very painful experiences. This resembles PTSD with reference to panic attacks. They develop a "fear of fear." They lose all their self-confidence with reference to their own mental health.

They will respond quickly to treatment with benzo-diazepines, but again due to concerns about benzodiaz-epines being addictive, etc., the psychiatrist is taught by his own profession to first treat panic attacks with SSRIs (antidepressants). There are no medications in the field of medicine as effective as benzodiazepines for the purpose they were intended for. In spite of some concerns about their use in the "addictive personality," there are no med-ications in the field of medicine with fewer side effects.

Unfortunately, I did not research Cochrane Studies with reference to treatment of panic attacks. But I do get many patients who have been treated for panic attacks with SSRIs unsuccessfully for years. On those rare occasions when SSRIs are effective, they probably should be used. I have had one patient with panic attacks who responded better to Paxil than to a benzodiazepine.

Xanax is a questionable benzodiazepine in so far as addiction and withdrawal possibilities are concerned, but Xanax is the "panic buster." Nothing will stop a panic attack as quickly as Xanax.

But, I will use longer-acting benzodiazepines such as clonazepam or diazepam trying to prevent the panic attacks. I may let them have just a few Xanax per month to stop breakthrough panic attacks. I have a high rate of success in trying to prevent panic attacks with longer acting benzodiazepines. When the patient has a few Xanax in a little aspirin case in his pocket, he regains his sense of self control. He loses his "fear of fear." He loses his fear of going crazy. Many of my patients will carry a few Xanax in their personal belongings for several years without ever taking one. Finally, they completely lose their fear of panic attacks and throw the Xanax away. It is very reassuring to them to carry a few Xanax even if they never have to use them.

Another immediate relief of some of the miseries of a panic attack can be accomplished by breathing into a paper bag. The patient is actually breathing too much when he feels like he cannot breathe. He depletes the normal amount of carbon dioxide in his blood which regulates the acid-base balance of his blood. This causes numbness around the mouth, numbness of the fingers, hyperreflexia of the muscles around the mouth and the hands. The patient can be educated about these things and regain some feeling of control of his panic attacks. This approach can ameliorate the pain of the panic attack if the patient can think well enough to follow these instructions. He retains some of his carbon dioxide by breathing into the paper bag while he is hyperventilating.

Thousands of dollars are spent in the emergency room evaluating these patients with reference to their heart and lungs. I had one patient in his 70s, who had had panic attacks since his 30s go to the emergency room 28 times in 30 days. This is very medically expensive. He just wanted a few Xanax to stop them. I trusted him and gave him a few Xanax. A few pennies replaced thousands of dollars in emergency room evaluations.

After the emergency room doctor has evaluated the patient to rule out medical problems, he will usually give the patient a few Xanax and a paper bag. Some patients will tell you that a panic attack is worse than a "heart attack."

Chapter 8

Psychosis

What is psychosis? All of us at times may distort reality to some extent as to the intentions of other people. When we are depressed, we may distort reality to some extent, but not in a bizarre way. But people with psychosis distort reality more severely and in a more bizarre way. Almost everyone who knows them is aware that they are mentally ill. Frequently you do not have to be a professional to make a diagnosis of psychosis. These serious distortions of reality occupy their minds so severely that they cannot "attend to business" such as bathing, preparing food, paying bills, and even sleeping. It can be very difficult to focus on any form of employment when the "voices" are constantly interrupting your train of thought. And a normal train of thought with logical conclusions may be impossible. Extreme depression or anxiety may accompany these serious thought disorders. With serious "thought blocking" these people may not be able to complete a sentence. They may believe that commentators on the television are talking about them (ideas of reference).

At times they are confused as to who they are and who their loved ones are. At times they feel as if they are standing outside of their body watching themselves. All of this makes normal social interactions extremely difficult and sometimes impossible.

Each of us throughout our lives believes in our own perceptions of reality around us. If someone becomes psychotic, they still believe in their own perception of reality. Certain experiences, such as shooting themselves due to command hallucinations, may cause "insight" so that they begin to accept the fact that not all of their perceptions of reality are correct. Perhaps taking antipsychotic medications that change their perception of reality causes "insight and improved judgment." Frequently society has to force them to take medications if they have no insight at all. This usually occurs when they are hospitalized because they have become a danger to themselves, a danger to others, or gravely disabled. Then, with the development of insight, they may take their medications voluntarily.

But after a while, thinking that they have recovered, they will discontinue their medications. About 99 percent of the time they relapse into psychosis when they stop taking their medications. This causes even more "insight." Due to these experiences, and with the passage of time, they become less of a danger to themselves or others because of their recognition that they need to take the medications. Sometimes they are very fearful of becoming psychotic again. Then they may take their medications routinely every day. Obviously they may get better now because they have truly developed important "insight."

They may become less disabled, but they are still disabled to the point that they cannot compete in a competitive workplace. There are people competing for simple work such as janitorial work. Psychotic people, even in fairly good remission, can rarely compete. Their emotional miseries will make it difficult for them to work competitively even while taking good antipsychotic medications. Some of the welfare money spent by the federal government goes to the worthy cause of keeping these people from starving and being homeless. The amount is usually 900 to 1100 dollars per month in Louisiana. I am not sure about other areas of the country. Many of them accidentally end up in prison where society will be taking care of them. A lot of harmless people end up in prison by accident due to poor judgment caused by mental illness or mild mental retardation. Do people sometimes con social welfare programs to get this money? Of course they do; but I know of many schizophrenic patients and bipolar patients who needed this help for several years before they finally got it. I have seen grown men cry when they got their first check.

The most common distortion of reality is auditory hallucinations. The second most common distortion of reality is visual hallucinations. Olfactory and tactile hallucinations are less common. Gustatory hallucinations are even more uncommon. These all involve our five senses.

The next most common distortion of reality is delusions. Delusions are fixed beliefs tightly held by the individual in spite of all evidence to the contrary. No one can reason with the individual using all kinds of evidence to the contrary. I never try to correct these delusional beliefs; the patient will think that I am calling him a liar and that will be the end of our doctor-patient relationship which is so important to their recovery. He will still believe what he believes no matter what anyone else in the world thinks. Some of these beliefs are extremely unlikely to be true, and everyone knows it but the individual.

Some of these people can "attend to business." Many years ago I took care of a small business owner in a VA hospital in Topeka, Kansas. He had gone for years believing that the federal government was trying to destroy him to keep him from revealing an act of malpractice. He stated that a needle had broken off in his shoulder muscle while in the service during the Second World War. If a pot fell out of a window while he was walking down the street, he would instantly blame it on the federal government. He went for years with this paranoid delusional belief before he finally ended up in a hospital.

Some of these delusional beliefs can be very bizarre. An example of a bizarre belief would be the schizophrenic patient who believes that a Martian implanted a chip in his brain that causes him to hear voices, or gives him commands as to what he should do. Most delusional beliefs concern being persecuted, being loved by someone, having magical powers, or distorted beliefs about their own body (somatic delusions). Some people who are not schizophrenic have paranoid delusions, but when the delusions are bizarre, they are always accompanied by multiple other distortions of reality. Then the diagnosis is always schizophrenia.

Illusions are not uncommon and not necessarily pathological. I may see a bush in the dark and think that it is a man. That would be an illusion. Another illusion is one that we've all experienced of driving down a road in the summer and seeing water on the pavement in the distance. As we keep driving, we all realize that that water is an illusion. Illusions are misinterpretations of what we actually see or hear.

Hallucinations are totally a product of the mind unrelated to reality. They do not misinterpret what they see; they see things that are not there. They hear things that no one else hears. Now we have discussed the most common distortions of reality: hallucinations, delusions, and illusions. The third one is not always pathological.

A schizophrenic patient is always psychotic. He or she is experiencing multiple distortions of reality. A bipolar patient can become psychotic while manic or while in the slowed down depression. A unipolar depressed person can become psychotic. The most common distortion of reality for these illnesses would be auditory hallucinations. A demented elderly person may become psychotic. For these people, visual hallucinations are slightly more common than auditory hallucinations. A person with delirium is psychotic due to withdrawal from a substance, often alcohol, or due to the effects of some medication. They are more prone to visual hallucinations. They frequently see small animals or small bugs running around the room or over their bodies, etc. A person with severe obsessive-compulsive disorder can become psychotic. The distortion of body image in eating disorders such as anorexia nervosa or bulimia might be considered of psychotic proportions. They tend to see themselves as obese even though they are actually starving. Certain hallucinogenic substances, such as LSD, PCP, mescaline, etc., nearly always cause visual hallucinations and possibly auditory hallucinations.

Another symptom of psychosis is disorganized thinking. Sometimes their speech is almost incomprehensible. Sometimes it is unrelated to the previous thought, or related in an illogical manner. Unrelated sentences would be considered "tangential thinking" or a "flight of ideas." Thoughts related in an illogical manner would be considered "loosening of associations." Some of our most humorous jokes from comedians are examples of "loosening of associations." Many disorganized schizophrenics can begin a train of thought but usually cannot finish it.

It is as if they lose their train of thought in midstream. This might be called "thought blocking." As they go from unfinished sentence to unfinished sentence, it is almost painful to watch them struggle to talk with you. The disorganized schizophrenic patient is lucky because they have a good prognosis for rapid response to antipsychotic medications.

The severely manic bipolar patient frequently has a "flight of ideas" where he jumps from topic to topic very rapidly. This is one of the hallmarks of mania along with a serious pressure of speech. Pressure of speech means that the patient talks rapidly and incessantly because the ideas are coming so fast to his mind. It is very hard for them to listen to anyone else. They will frequently answer my questions before I can ask them.

I have one story to tell that illustrates a defect in the thinking of a schizophrenic patient. I do not have a quick way of summarizing this problem. A certain woman in Southern California in the 1970s was always going to see physicians about a pain in her abdomen which no one could find any cause for. I was asked to see the patient in consultation regarding her emotional state. She seemed quite normal during the first part of the interview. There was no "weirdness" of affect. She gave no evidence of any emotional problems. But somehow I obtained an old hospital chart concerning a previous admission to the hospital for a similar problem. During that hospitalization she simply got out of bed and walked out of the second story window of her room. She broke bones in her feet. I was thinking that she might have been suicidal. I ask her why she walked out of the second story window. She replied that she did not have the money to pay her hospital bill. This is a dramatic example of the abnormal thinking of a schizophrenic patient. When I heard that story, her diagnosis became obvious.

Schizophrenia is the classical illness described as psychosis. Auditory hallucinations are nearly always present. These hallucinations are frequently very derogatory. Sometimes they have command hallucinations telling them to commit *hara-kiri* with a knife. Sometimes they command the patient to drown himself. Sometimes they just make a constant running comment on his every move and every thought.

Many years ago a schizophrenic patient told me that there were three men following him around making comments about the way he walked, or about the way his "balls" hang down, etc. "Do you notice the way his toes turn out?" I cannot remember the total conversation of the three men who were talking about him — but you get the idea. Their comments were very derogatory, and I am hesitant to repeat many of them in this book. Very rarely the voices may tell him to kill someone else — but this must be extremely rare. I have never had a schizophrenic patient tell me that the voices were telling him to kill someone else. I now think of one exception, a man who killed his parents. He was in prison at the time I treated him. Usually the voices are destructive towards himself.

One of my patients jumped overboard from a large boat somewhere south of the equator to the west of South America. The voices told him that if he did not jump overboard, they would "turn him inside out through his ass hole."

One of my patients told me that at age 29 he was driving down the highway and begin to hear the voices. He had a delivery job at that time. Ten years later, age 39, he was still hearing the voices. They just came out of nowhere and never stopped. They were very emotionally disturbing to him. He could hardly stand it. It was very hard for him to continue working. He finally went on disability due to the constant voices. He tried to ignore them. That is very hard to do. While talking to me and trying to carry on a conversation with me, he could not help but try to listen to the voices at the same time to see what they were saying. His appearance did not reveal his illness.

Some patients have good insight that the voices are not real, or at least that no one else hears them. Other patients do not have this insight. They will be looking around the room while talking with me, trying to see where the voices are coming from. They may also have various delusional beliefs at the same time.

Years ago, when Freud was still very influential, we

believed that paranoid delusional beliefs were due to repressed or unrecognized homosexual feelings. I did hospitalize a man many years ago in a psychiatric unit early one morning. When I went back to see him at noon, he ran up to me and told me that the psychiatric unit was full of "queers." He was more than willing to point them out to me. I can't help but believe that he was projecting his own inner repressed feelings onto these other men. That is my Freudian education from the 1950s influencing my thinking. Or, could he simply have a delusional belief for some unknown reason that all of these men were in love with him? This man was not very frightening. Even though his view of reality was very different from mine, he could confide in me as to what he was thinking and feeling.

A severely paranoid schizophrenic patient, untreated, can be very frightening and threatening. You know that they want you to stay at a distance. They will talk to you if you keep the distance of about 10 feet. They will not let you get any closer. Even though they are very threatening, like a barking dog, I feel sure they must have a great deal of fear also. Consequently I give them that 10 feet of space while I'm talking with them. After successful medication, which can be challenging, they will invite you into their room, sit down close to you, and carry on an extremely friendly and socially sensitive conversation. The difference is stunning between an unmedicated paranoid schizophrenic and a properly medicated paranoid schizo-phrenic. My personal experience is that the dosages of medication had to be high to do this. My best experi-ence was with a combination of about 40 mg of Haldol and 40 mg of Prolixin. These are older antipsychotics not frequently used today. And most psychiatrists would consider these dosages to be rather large, especially when combined with each other. But in my experience, it took a large amount of antipsychotic medication to bring about this rather miraculous change.

The typical onset of schizophrenia is between ages seventeen and 25, but it can start in their 30s rarely. Apparently bizarre behavior or non-socially appropriate behavior in the high school setting with early use of mind altering substances, depression, etc. can predict that that individual may become schizophrenic. Also many schizo-phrenic patients experienced depression before they began to have auditory hallucinations. And many schizophrenic patients complain of severe anxiety.

Leaders in the field of psychiatry are very interested in learning how to predict who will become schizophrenic so that they can begin medication to avoid the onset of the illness. Also it is most important that the first episode of schizophrenia be treated very adequately and com-pletely and followed with antipsychotic medications for some prolonged period of time to avoid a second episode. Sometimes this approach is successful. It is wonderful if they never have a second episode. So adequate treatment of the first episode is mandatory. But for most schizophrenic patients it is a lifelong illness. Insight may increase. They may decide to continue their medications as prescribed and never stop them. Some schizophrenic patients learn the hard way to be very religious about taking their medications. They do not want to get sick again. It is a frightening experience.

I followed one wonderful person who was schizophrenic for 14 years. I used one of the older medications called first-generation antipsychotics to differentiate from second-generation antipsychotics more commonly used today. I had him on a rather constant dose of medication, but at times I had to increase it slightly due to some increased stress such as getting a new roommate. He attempted to work, but any stressor could make him very anxious, and I knew that when he became anxious that the voices were about to return. One job he attempted to do in a hot factory put him in the emergency room packed in ice with a fan blowing on him to reduce his core temperature. Most of the antipsychotic medications, if not all, interferes with our temperature regulating mechanisms of the body such as shivering or sweating, etc. Once they have a very severe heatstroke, they are much more likely to have another one. That experience seems to leave some permanent alterations in their temperature regulating mechanisms. If he ever reads this book, I want to give him my apologies for deserting him back in 1980 and my best wishes for his current life.

I followed many patients with schizophrenia for six to eight years at least. Medication control for them was similar to the first patient I have mentioned. A good doctor-patient relationship is essential to have this kind of medication compliance from the patient.

Sometimes the parents will allow a schizophrenic patient to stay at home with them indefinitely. They know this child is different from their other children. Many times they will never get married, but this is not always true. Some of them leave home and attempt marriage. Marital life is usually rocky and unsuccessful. They often become very withdrawn and despondent. Their affect is often described as blunted, flat, or bizarre. They may not pay much attention to their cleanliness, dress, and personal appearance in general. They usually avoid other people and other people avoid them.

Sometimes following successful treatment with medication, they are able to "attend to business." This is what one of my schizophrenic patients said to me. He was of moderate disability. With medication he could pay his bills, take a bath, clean his clothes, cook some, etc. When his mind was full of distracting thoughts, unrelated to reality, he could not "attend to business."

We are beginning to realize that the blunting of affect and other" negative symptoms" of schizophrenia might be helped by antidepressants. Perhaps a benzodiazepine can be very helpful for anxiety. I've seen this on many occasions. But, the underlying antipsychotic medication must be continued at the same time. The first second-generation antipsychotic, Risperdal, was touted to be better at diminishing negative symptoms than the older first-generation antipsychotics such as Thorazine, Stelazine, Prolixin, Haldol, etc. I am not sure that this has turned out to be a significant observation. Some of the newer antipsychotics such as Seroquel (quetiapine) and Zyprexa (olanzapine) have more pronounced negative metabolic effects such as weight gain, increased cholesterol, etc. Geodon (ziprasidone) does not have these negative metabolic side effects usually, but it often will not stop the voices. I've only mentioned a few of the newer medications.

It is commonly believed that the older medications caused more extrapyramidal symptoms such as restlessness, muscle contractions,and outright parkinsonism. These can be treated and medication can be continued. The most dreaded one was persistent tardive dyskinesia. This was a strange repetitive movement around the tongue, mouth or arms that never went away. Notice the word persistent. Tardive dyskinesia might not be persistent. Muscle dystonias can also be persistent. When the newer drugs came out, a lot of money was at stake in their promotion by the pharmaceutical industry. I began to hear how frequent persistent tardive dyskinesia was due to the older medications. "The word was" that 25 percent of patients who were on the older antipsychotics for any period of time would develop persistent tardive dyskinesia. I never had a case of tardive dyskinesia with the older drugs in years gone by, but recently, just days before publishing this book, I did have a case of tardive dyskinesia involving a woman taking fluphenazine 1 mg two times per day, an extremely low dosage. From this viewpoint, I suppose I was just very lucky. But I have seen it with two of the newer drugs, Risperdal and Abilify. In fact, I've seen it more often with the newer drugs than the older drugs.

Theoretically, from a pharmacological viewpoint, the older drugs should cause more persistent tardive dyskinesia than the newer drugs. But I just have not personally seen it — I have seen the opposite. It is certainly hard for me to believe that the older drugs will cause tardive dyskinesia in 25 percent of the patients who take them for any length of time. And many younger psychiatrists believe this to be true. That is just not my experience with them. And I think it would be a mistake in the treatment of some patients to always avoid the first-generation antipsychotics because of the possibility of tardive dyskinesia. To keep this side effect in mind is one thing; to completely shun them would be an unfortunate loss of an effective treatment of schizophrenia. And some of the leaders in psychiatry, while lecturing to large audiences, will exclude the use of first-generation antipsychotics because of the possibility of tardive dyskinesia. I suppose, in the last sentence or two, I'm addressing my fellow psychiatrists rather than the general public. But I had hoped to address this book to the general public. Obviously my viewpoint on this matter is debatable; but 25 percent is a very large percentage. I have no way of knowing for sure, but I might believe that 5 percent, maybe even 10 percent, of patients who are on the older first-generation antipsychotics for many years will develop permanent tardive dyskinesia consisting of repetitive movements of the tongue or lips or upper extremities. But these older antipsychotics did not cause as much weight gain or increased cholesterol or adult onset diabetes, etc. And when the "chips are down," low dosages of the older antipsychotics added to the newer ones may stop auditory hallucinations when all else is failing.

I have to make some comments about my own personal experiences with schizophrenia. I started my residency in psychiatry at the VA hospital in Topeka, Kansas, very much affiliated with the Menninger School of Psychiatry, in 1959. There were 1000 psychiatric beds at the VA hospital and there were 1000 psychiatric beds at Topeka State Hospital. The Menninger brothers had been very influential in reforming the old Topeka State Hospital from a rather primitive approach to mental illness to a much more humane approach. There were 15 residents in each class at each hospital. This was a total of 90 residents. At that time the US government wanted to increase the number of practicing psychiatrists because Will Menninger had convinced the government that there was an extreme shortage of psychiatrists during the Second World War.

I had 20 schizophrenic patients who had been in the hospital since the Second World War. This was 1959. Most of them had never received any of the new antipsychotic medications which were just coming into psychiatric practice. They were definitely chronic schizophrenics. They all smoked heavily, which is typical of schizophrenic patients. Their fingernails were yellow. One of the patients was hebephrenic. This is a type of schizophrenia which causes the patient to giggle continuously. Eye contact is almost nonexistent. They always have their head down, in a corner, giggling. Hebephrenia is no longer even mentioned in the DSM V or the DSM-IV. This particular hebephrenia patient was told that he had an illness (probably a bulging inguinal hernia) that required surgery. He suddenly changed personalities and begin to "attend to business." He ask all of the appropriate questions about possible outcomes with surgery and without surgery. He ask all the appropriate questions concerning complications of surgery. He decided to have the surgery. Prior to surgery and for two or three weeks after surgery his affect was completely normal. Then he began to exhibit symptoms of hebephrenia again. This very much puzzled a beginning resident. I have never really been sure how to understand this.

I think under serious stress a schizophrenic patient can briefly rise to the occasion and perform normally, possibly related to some biochemical change such as increased norepinephrine in the brain due to the stress? I really have no certainty of the reason.

Years ago the story was told that during the Second World War the psychiatric patients, probably schizophrenics, were released from a mental institution in France. They disappeared into the countryside and were never hospitalized again. That is hard for me to believe, but I can believe that they rose to the occasion initially when released from the hospital into the countryside to survive as best they could.

There were 20 patients full of rage, extremely prone to violence, in another ward of the VA hospital I trained in. They all voluntarily wore leather cuffs around their wrist so that they would not harm someone in a reflex manner. They could get their hands out of the cuffs, but then they would voluntarily put them back into the cuffs.

One day I was talking to another patient in that unit leaning against the wall. A different patient came up to me asking for a "light." I was intent on my conversation and put my hand out to touch his shoulder to wait a minute. Instantly he kicked me in the buttocks. It was a reflex when I touched him. Patients like these are never seen today. They've all been treated with antipsy-chotic medications which began to come into existence in 1955 and have increased in number over the last 58 to 60 years. Untreated chronic schizophrenics are now non-existent.

DSM IV and DSM V lists several types of schizo-phrenia. I stated at the beginning of this book that this is not a textbook of psychiatry. I will not attempt to enu-merate the various types of schizophrenia. The diagnosis is usually based on the most prominent symptoms.

One classical type, different from all the rest, prob-ably should be mentioned. The catatonic patient is fro-zen in space. I have been taught that he has a delusional belief that if he moves he will destroy the world. He may not eat or sleep or urinate for prolonged periods of time. They simply will not respond in any way when someone approaches them. Not even their eyes move. They are always staring straight ahead into space. Today a catatonic patient would probably be treated in an intensive care unit with intravenous Ativan (lorazepam), a benzodiazepine, until he was mobile and could partake of food, sleep, etc. I personally have seen only a few catatonic individuals. I only mention them because they are strikingly different from other schizophrenic patients. They may stand with their arms extended in front of them. If you raise one of their arms, they will hold it in place indefinitely. This is referred to as "waxy flexibility." They do not talk. They stare straight ahead. They do not move their eyes. They will not respond in any way to your questions. Their faces are expressionless.

In general, about six or seven percent of all schizophrenic patients will successfully commit suicide. About 20 percent will make attempts.

As I mentioned earlier, people with severe unipolar depression can become psychotic. They usually begin to hear voices which are extremely critical of them, even using very insulting language to the patient. They will rationalize suicide as the only appropriate action to take. They can work incessantly to convince the patient to commit suicide. It is most common of all to tell the patient how worthless they are. These accusations are not built on any facts whatsoever. I theorize that the voices are the inner critic changing from thoughts to auditory hallucinations. I have talked about the inner critic at length in another chapter. This may not fully describe the hallucinations of psychotic unipolar depression, but it almost does. These people had a similar type of thinking generated by their inner critic before they began to hear voices.

I cannot really differentiate the psychotic thinking of a Bipolar I slowed down depression from the psychotic thinking of the unipolar depression. Everything I said in the above paragraph about unipolar depressed psychotic thinking would apply equally to the bipolar depression.

It is as if the thoughts generated by their inner critic have become auditory hallucinations.

One of the most important things to know about bipolar disorder is that it is the number one cause of suicide. And I'm sure they often are psychotic when they do it. Three brilliant, successful, handsome, young psychiatrists I have known committed suicide. As the saying goes, "they had absolutely everything going for them." They were all admired by their peers. Each of their suicides was almost unbelievable to their peers. We could not understand it. I am sure they were all bipolar. Bipolar disorder is the number one killer among the various mental illnesses.

Visual hallucinations are very common in early dementia; sometimes they might even be the presenting symptom. Of course the dementia was present first, but not yet diagnosed. The very last thing to change with dementia is their social facade. Very successful people can carry on a charming conversation with you, but they do not have the slightest idea what the year is. They may be off by 30 years. They cannot find the restroom which is just behind them. But they are still charming socially. At least ask the date when talking with these people. Such rudimentary facts are more diagnostic than social charm.

I had a patient who was looking out the second story window of his home and shooting a rifle at people who were stealing his tools from his workshop next to his garage. Family members ask him what he was shooting at? He told them. The locks to the tool shed were all in place. There was no evidence whatsoever that anyone there was carrying off his tools. This is a dramatic example of visual hallucinations in early dementia. They can also have auditory hallucinations sometimes.

The most common change with dementia, of a psychotic nature, is paranoid delusions. They become distrustful of their loved ones if their loved ones make any attempt to curtail their activities for their own safety and well-being. In fact, paranoid thinking is just under the surface in nearly all people who are losing their mental abilities. Slight paranoia, not considered psychotic, abounds in nearly all of us. It is no wonder that paranoia becomes more serious as dementia develops. Due to paranoia, and sometimes grandiosity, the demented patient may strike out at caregivers who are insolent enough to try to tell them when to eat breakfast, bath, etc.

Using a very low-dose of an antipsychotic medication can be very helpful for this problem. There is a black box warning from the FDA on all antipsychotic medications that they may cause earlier deaths in these people for a myriad of causes. They do not say exactly why these antipsychotic medications cause earlier death, but research has shown they do. But these people definitely need minimal amounts of antipsychotic medications so that they can be taken care of appropriately. And sedation is not what I am talking about. We do not want the patient to be over sedated by these medications. And all of these medications have side effects which must be watched for. But doesn't it stand to reason that when an elderly person becomes demented, their death will be hastened by the dementia, perhaps unrelated to the antipsychotic medication. They simply cannot look after themselves as well as the elderly who are not demented. Alzheimer's disease in itself leads slowly to death.

Small bugs and small animals crawling on them or around them is classic for delirium. I had one patient who loved to party to excess. He told me that one morning he woke up in a hotel room and saw mice coming in and out through the keyhole. He quit drinking entirely. This scared him badly. As the years went by, he became an outstanding citizen of the community he lived in. This was delirium due to heavy drinking, but delirium usually occurs during withdrawal from heavy drinking.

I saw a six-year-old boy having visual hallucinations (delirium) due to an intravenous antibiotic given by his surgeon following surgery. That surgeon had given that same antibiotic hundreds of times without any problems. But the literature revealed that on rare occasion this antibiotic, given intravenously, can cause visual hallucinations. Sudden withdrawal from certain medications can cause delirium. This is especially true if medication caused some degree of sedation which the body has adapted to.

Rarely people with serious obsessive-compulsive disorders can become psychotic. I once treated a lady who was having extremely intrusive disturbing thoughts about something unthinkably bad, such as having some sort of sexual interaction with Jesus. For a religious woman, you can imagine how distasteful these intrusive thoughts were. This patient would not tell me any details about her thoughts. They were too distasteful for her to talk about. I interpret these intrusive thoughts as being part of her serious obsessive-compulsive illness. They were the obsessive thoughts. She also had certain compulsive behaviors to cope with these thoughts. She would make coffee repeatedly, pour it out, and make it again. In obsessive compulsive illness there is always an obsession followed by compulsive behavior. Psychiatric textbooks do state that there can be a psychotic element to serious obsessive-compulsive disorders, and that is my experience also on several occasions. These intrusive thoughts can be muted or eliminated by antipsychotic medications. This paragraph is not intended to be a comprehensive discussion of obsessive-compulsive disorders. I only intended to point out that obsessive-compulsive disorders can have a psychotic element.

I have not treated many people with anorexia nervosa or bulimia. As most of you know, people with anorexia nervosa see themselves as obese and consequently will not eat adequately to maintain a healthy body weight. They develop many serious health problems simply because they will not eat. In the early stages, when they are physically able, they may exercise extensively to lose weight. They eventually become bedridden skeletons, but they will not eat because they see themselves as obese. I, and many other psychiatrists, will refer these patients to other psychiatrists and other mental health workers who specialize in treating this illness. They are exceedingly difficult to treat successfully. Their view of their bodies as obese is obviously a distortion of reality, and under my definition given earlier in this chapter, they would have to be considered psychotic.

Bulimia is an illness where people eat excessive amounts of food and then cause themselves to vomit to maintain a more ideal weight. As far as I know, they do not have an unrealistic view of their bodies. Even though they do have an illness, they are not psychotic.

Certain hallucinogenic substances such as LSD, PCP, Mescaline nearly always cause visual hallucinations and possibly auditory hallucinations. In my opinion these substances cause a temporary psychosis. I will never forget the story of a young man exposed to LSD sitting on a grassy knoll close to downtown Los Angeles where many of the freeways coming from East and West and North and South cross. He was in the middle of it all in a psychotic state of mind. I do not remember how he managed to get himself to that location while he was psychotic. I can only imagine the fear and anxiety he was experiencing. This paragraph is in no way an attempt to give a scholarly presentation concerning hallucinogenic substances. But I will say in passing that I have seen patients exposed to PCP who developed states of psychosis which lasted as long as six or seven years.

One particular patient had been a successful businessman before taking PCP (phencyclidine). Six or seven years later he was working as a chef when I met him, but he was still experiencing auditory hallucinations. He had good insight as to what his problem was, but he had to take antipsychotic medications to function.

Treatment of psychosis is a complex issue which I have touched upon slightly in passing. But I consider the medications involved too complex for this book. Always obtain professional help from a trained psychiatrist in coping with any psychosis. Medication has to be the "backbone" of treatment for any psychosis.

Chapter 9

ATTENTION DEFICIT HYPERACTIVITY DISORDER

It is not uncommon for children to be hyperactive and easily distractible early in their life before age six. Common sense would tell us that a few children might exhibit these behaviors beyond age six, but the vast majority of children will be able to go to kindergarten and later the first grade and behave in an age-appropriate manner. But unfortunately, good research has shown for several years now that six to eight percent of children all over the world have this problem referred to as ADHD or ADD.

I once heard a psychiatrist on television stating that this problem was peculiar to the United States and does not happen in England or Germany, etc. This is simply misleading and untruthful. There are some people in the United States who would like to believe that this is not a real mental illness. Even a rare schoolteacher has made comments to me along those lines. The implication is that their behavior is a product of inadequate parenting involving setting proper limits among other things. As the years pass, more and more people have come to realize that this is a mental illness that deserves proper recognition and treatment, not increased punishments or limit setting. It is now recognized by knowledgeable mental health professionals that a large percentage of people with this problem will require treatment during their adult lives for ADHD or ADD, and that 20 to 25 percent of these adults will exhibit symptoms of generalized anxiety disorder, or depression, or bipolar disorder. Recent research suggests that children may have genetics for ADHD or bipolar disorder. Unfortunately some children will have the genetics for both. In this case, psychiatrists usually treat the bipolar disorder first and the ADHD symptoms second. Later we will discuss how psychiatrists attempt to differentiate ADHD from bipolar mania.

The easiest time to make the diagnosis of ADHD is around age five through seven. When a parent would bring a child to see me in this age group, I could see in a moment what the diagnosis was. The child would exhibit a whirlwind of activity running all over my office, into the drawers of my desk, perhaps crawling up on my desk, or examining objects on my desk. In self-defense I would quickly give them something to do. The easiest thing was to hand them a tablet of drawing paper with crayons and request that they draw something for me. They would quickly go to work on this project to avoid "boredom." Then the mother and schoolteachers would give me the confirming history that I needed to make the diagnosis. The mother would say, for example, that she has five children. This child is just different from her other four children. The parenting skills, love, limit setting, perhaps punishment were all administered in the same manner to all five children. Four children responded beautifully. This fifth child was just different. The fifth child with ADHD was jumping off the refrigerator, jumping off couches, talking incessantly, unable to sit at the table for a meal, unable to follow simple directions. They were so quickly distracted by other stimuli that following simple directions was very difficult. Some of them could not go to sleep until after midnight. For some of them sleep was not a problem. But those children who could not go to sleep until after midnight were exhausting for the parents. They could not follow the rules in kindergarten and they could not follow the rules in the first grade. They could not remain in their seats; they could not stop talking at inappropriate times; they could not listen to the teacher; if they knew the answer to a question, they could not wait to be called upon; they could not wait in line at the cafeteria, etc.

Most children with this problem will make barely passing grades, or perhaps fail. I did have a child or two so brilliant that they could make excellent grades even though they appeared to not be listening. All of these children receive a great deal of negative feedback. This leads to strong feelings of inadequacy and shame and guilt. As the years pass they will begin to associate with other "losers." These are the children who grow up and try mind altering substances usually referred to as "drugs," drop out of school, get in more trouble, and receive more negative feedback. It is a vicious cycle for all involved. This may be the reason that ADHD children treated with stimulants are less likely to abuse drugs in later years than those children who go untreated. There is good research to support the above statement.

And remember, for some reason stimulants are calming or sedating for these children and do not stimulate them as they would normal children. That is why that ADHD children receiving too large a dose of stimulant medication may appear over sedated. Some mothers, more than one, have said to me, "I do not want you to give my son any of that Ritalin and make him a zombie like my nephew." I would assume that the nephew was overmedicated.

Children with attention deficit disorder (ADD), but not hyperactivity (ADHD), are usually not diagnosed until they are a little older. They may not make very good grades because they cannot listen to the teacher, but they do not cause problems in the classroom like ADHD children. Both types can only focus on something they are very interested in.

I forgot to point out that by age 12, approximately,

a child with ADHD has developed adequate self-control to sit in my office talking with me for perhaps 45 minutes without exhibiting hyperactivity or impulsivity. Their diagnosis is more difficult. Without the hyperactivity shown in earlier years, my diagnosis has to be made based on what the child tells me and what the parent and schoolteachers tell me. This of course is also true of adults with these problems. I have to base my diagnosis on past history, although there are sophisticated test administered by psychologist which can help confirm the diagnosis during adult years. A very few cases of ADHD in adults did not originate during childhood. I cannot explain this. Sometimes head trauma can cause either bipolar disorder or ADHD.

My theory is that they are experiencing an inner misery which is like severe boredom. Most of us are very busy and do not have time to be bored. But boredom is a miserable state. I hypothesize that some elderly people with mild to moderate dementia in nursing homes simply end their lives by stopping their intake of food and water. They simply go into a coma and die out of boredom. When you cannot do anything due to dementia, cannot recognize the people you eat lunch with, cannot get involved with anyone else, cannot understand what is happening on television, then boredom is inevitable.

One time I played hooky by telling my mother that I was ill. We did not have television in those days. She made me stay in bed all day with nothing to do. I was extremely bored. The next morning, I jumped out of bed, told her that I was miraculously cured, and begged to go back to school. I hypothesize that boredom is horrible and I hypothesize that these children are indescribably bored. The children will tell me they are bored. The mother will tell me that they are always bored or saying that they are bored. I have seen little children scream in protest when the mother takes some electronic gadget away from them that is entertaining to them. If something is entertaining to them, they are often prone to over focus on that to the exclusion of everything else. They are also very impulsive as I've already described above. This may be a product of boredom. I have adult patients who like to ride motorcycles at very high speeds, jump off of high cliffs into the ocean, all of which causes "adrenaline rushes." Are they bored? I am not sure, but it is an interesting question. For whatever it is worth, I believe these children with ADHD or ADD are unutterably bored.

Mothers worry about what the long term effects of stimulants may be on their children. They will not give the stimulants on weekends because they are not in school. They may not give the stimulants during the summer months. Sometimes they will give the stimulants year around because they cannot tolerate the behavior of the children when they are unmedicated. And some children will request that they receive their stimulant all of the time because they are much happier taking the stimulant rather than being severely bored. In my opinion, treatment of these two illnesses is not just so that the child can be successful in school; the treatment is for a type of mental illness and success in school is simply a byproduct of treatment for this mental illness.

It is difficult to explain how the psychiatrists attempt to differentiate ADHD from Bipolar Disorder. First I must admit that this can be difficult to do, and during initial consultations the proper diagnosis may be missed. Please give the psychiatrist a little time to get the right diagnosis. At worst, the final scenario could be that the psychiatrist makes the right diagnosis based on the child's response to medication.

Both illnesses can exhibit hyperactivity, impulsivity, etc, but a few aspects of bipolar disorder might help us to make the right diagnosis. For one thing, bipolar disorder may be episodic lasting a few days or a few weeks or even months, but there will be periods of time when the child is normal in feelings and behavior. Bipolar disorder is usually episodic. ADHD is not episodic; these children have their problem 24 hours a day, 7 days a week without relief.

Bipolar children may have episodes of rage which I think exceeds ADHD anger. Some psychiatrists believe that bipolar children must exhibit some aspects of euphoria, gross overestimation of their abilities, and invincibility. I believe that some children with bipolar disorder exhibit rage, etc., but not necessarily euphoria or overestimation of their abilities. I also believe that many adults with bipolar mania do not exhibit euphoria or overestimation of themselves, but simply rage, depression, anxiety, paranoia, etc. They are diagnosed as having mixed mania. I have discussed this more thoroughly in the chapter on bipolar disorder. In a nutshell, I believe that some bipolar adults and children never exhibit any type of euphoria thought by many to be absolutely essential to make a diagnosis of mania.

An immense amount of research money is being spent to discover the neuroanatomical and neurochemical basis for this disorder. Many theories are being offered as a result of this extensive research. I would like to refer the reader to "Stahl's Essential Psychopharmacology" fourth edition published in 2013. A very simple summary would be to say that the disorder involves a problem with dopamine and norepinephrine in the brain. The stimulants that are used to treat this disorder cause more norepinephrine and dopamine in the brain.

There are many degrees of severity of ADHD. One of the worst examples would be a mother who spent almost two hours daily working with a child, perhaps age 11, to complete homework that should have taken only 15 to 30 minutes. The child could not focus on the task without constant encouragement from the mother. Quite a few of these people will finish high school with low passing grades. Some will find work which accommodates their illness; rarely their illness may be an advantage in certain types of work. Marriages can be strained. Finishing four years of college will be a monumental task. And after finishing college, the man or woman with untreated ADHD or ADD may not be able to do the work they have been educated for because of their neurological problem.

Sometimes I have had great difficulty in making the proper diagnosis. I had one girl about age 11 who always seemed to me to be depressed. The mother always appeared overly critical and angry. Unfortunately, I treated this young girl for depression for at least a year. Then during one session, it was mentioned that she needed to be in a classroom by herself during testing because of her easy distractibility. It is not unusual that ADHD children need to be alone during testing. Sometimes they are placed at the front of the classroom so that they may be able to more easily focus on what the teacher says. Suddenly I realized that this girl might have ADHD. She never exhibited any hyperactivity in my office. She never mentioned boredom. When I started a stimulant, her performance in school was greatly enhanced and her depression totally disappeared. I did not see her very often after that. When I did, she was always happy and even her mother was smiling.

A large amount of research over the years has been conducted to find the long-range deleterious effects of stimulants on these children. Fortunately, so far, nothing at all has been found. Stimulants are probably one of the safest drugs given by the medical profession, but they nearly always cause decreased appetite.

A few immediate side effects of importance are possible. Dysrhythmias could develop if the child has some anatomical cardiac abnormality or abnormalities of the EKG. Approximately 2005, the American Heart Association and the American Association of Cardiologist issued a statement that all children, about to be started on a stimulant, should have a thorough cardiac history taken including an EKG.

In addition to a cardiac evaluation, some psychiatrists would worry about worsening seizures. Some neurologists don't worry about this at all. If they have seizures, I always consult their neurologist before prescribing stimulants. Many times they will tell me not to worry about it.

Stimulants could increase tics; I find this rare but definitely possible. There is relatively new research indicating that alpha-2 agonist, such as clonidine, when administered with the stimulant, may prevent tics.

All children should have follow-up concerning blood pressure and pulse rate after being prescribed a stimulant. On a few occasions I have found this to be a problem. On occasion I have changed the child from one type of stimulant to another type to solve this problem. Usually this treatment has been successful.

Stimulants often decrease the appetite of these

children and stunt growth. I often administered a medication that would help with sleep and increase appetite when needed. There is some research to suggest that over the following years the child will catch up in their growth, but I would feel more comfortable doing something to increase their appetite when needed while prescribing a stimulant. Decreased appetite is the most frequent side effect of stimulants.

One boy came to me already on stimulants only weighing about 84 pounds. About the third or fourth interview, I got the history that at one time he had weighed about 105 pounds. I cut the stimulant down in dosage. His appetite picked up and he grew rapidly attaining good height and all the characteristics of a developing adult male about age 14 or 15.

What are these stimulants? Simply put, there are two families of stimulants. The first one discovered in the 1930s was Dexedrine (dextroamphetamine). The second one discovered in the 1960s was Ritalin (methylphenidate). So, we have two families of stimulants.

Each family has received modifications so that there are multiple forms of these stimulants, but in the final analysis only two families. Methylphenidate has a modification called desmethylphenidate (Focalin) which is about 1 1/2 times as strong as Ritalin. Several extended release forms of Ritalin have been developed so that theoretically the child has to take medication only one time per day rather than three times per day. Sometimes these extended release forms do not take effect for two or three hours. The child can get in a lot of trouble on the school bus going to school before these extended-release forms take effect. And usually they will need a top up dose around 2 p.m. daily because I find that the extended-release forms do not last 12 hours as advertised. Ritalin (methylphenidate), not extended-release, takes effect in 30 minutes and lasts four or five hours. If you're watching a young child, you can see an immediate change in their behavior. It is miraculous. I like these immediate release forms because I know pretty much what to expect from them. The child may have to take the immediate release form three times per day to cover 12 or 14 hours. Some children do well with the extended-release forms, and parents often prefer the extended-release. But remember, most of these children in my experience will need a smaller dose of some form around 2 p.m. daily. The extended-release form never last 12 hours as advertised.

Dextroamphetamine also has been modified multiple times and newer and probably more effective versions have been developed. The most frequently used is Adderall (amphetamine salts) which includes the original dextro-amphetamine, but also amphetamine, and possibly levo-amphetamine. I am not sure about the levoamphetamine, but it does include at least three amphetamine salts which seem to be preferred by most patients in comparison to the original dextroamphetamine (Dexedrine). Adderall has also been modified so that several extended-release forms are available. The exact form of Adderall which is most advantageous for a child or adult must be found through trials of the medications searching for the one which works best for that patient. I will not give exact dosages, but I always start with the lowest dose and increase it gradually over a period of several weeks or even a month or so until the parents, school teachers, or the older patients themselves tell me that that dosage is best for them. I do not have to be stingy about this controlled substance. I start low and they tell me when to stop. I had a 65-year-old adult male weighing approximately 250 pounds. I started him on a very low dose of Ritalin that I might have given to a six-year-old child. He said "stop." The low-dose was all he needed.

Another form of Dexedrine (dextroamphetamine) has been developed called Vyvanse (lisdexamfetamine). This is not an extremely new drug, but it is newer than Adderall or Ritalin. It is not a stimulant in itself, but rather a prodrug which is cleaved in the stomach into the active compounds of dextroamphetamine and free L-lysine. So it is not a stimulant until after it is swallowed. The experience I have with Vyvanse leads me to believe that it is the one stimulant which may last a whole day. I have a rare patient that may need a top up dose, but not often. As usual, I start on the lowest dose and increase gradually until everyone concerned tells me that I have reached the proper dose. I do not dose by weight with any of these stimulants although, the manufacturers recommend not exceeding certain dosages based on weight. I do follow these recommendations for the most part. Decreased appetite or lack of weight gain will influence my dosage. Other side effects may limit my dosage. Vyvanse seems to have a smoother onset and be effective for longer duration. It is very popular among those who can afford it. It is more expensive.

Another reason to prescribe Vyvanse when possible is that it is a prodrug. It is not a stimulant that can be snorted or injected intravenously. It must be swallowed into the stomach before becoming a stimulant. An addict would have no use for this drug. They are going to request Adderall at the highest dose possible.

I do hope that I have convinced you that ADHD and ADD are serious neurological illnesses for which there is good treatment. Everyone, parents and older patients, should persistently seek good treatment until they have found it.

Unfortunately, some psychiatrists are overly concerned that an adult patient is actually an addict seeking stimulants to feed their addiction. Of course, this rarely happens, but it is unfortunate when this over concern prevents someone with ADHD or ADD from getting the treatment they desperately need. The addict would prefer "speed" (methamphetamine) (called by various street names) to the drugs I am prescribing. Methamphetamine is considerably more effective for the addicts needs. I do my best to never give stimulants to an addict, but I am only human. Frequently someone who is addicted to a substance is a genius at obtaining it through the proper lies. There are extremely good questionnaires to give to adult patients to identify ADHD, but they could simply answer in the positive to all these questions. I think it is probably impossible to be perfectly accurate clinically in the diagnosis of adult ADHD. History from their parents about their childhood could be very helpful. And sophisticated psychological testing by a psychologist could be very beneficial.

There are a few medical conditions that partially or completely preclude the use of stimulants. These are glaucoma, hyperthyroidism, severe anxiety, hypertension, and Raynaud's phenomenon. One type of medication, MAOI inhibitors, completely precludes the use of stimulants.

Chapter 10

BORDERLINE PERSONALITY DISORDER

I have treated multiple borderline personalities, but not nearly enough to consider myself an expert. The most important source of information for me, and I can strongly recommend it to everyone else, including professionals, is "Borderline Personality Disorder — A Multidimensional Approach" by Joel Paris, MD. This book has approximately 400 references, largely the work of other psychiatrists, several of which had devoted their lives exclusively to the treatment of borderline personality disorders. This book is packed with information concerning the diagnosis and possible treatments of this type of emotional illness. Dr. Paris is a Professor, Department of Psychiatry, McGill University and Research Associate, Department of Psychiatry, Jewish General Hospital. I will try to condense this book into a few salient points to keep in mind with reference to the diagnosis and treatment of this emotional illness. Such a condensation inherently has risk. For anyone who needs more information, or simply desires more information, please read Dr. Paris' book for yourself. Anyone who thinks they have this problem, possibly diagnosed by their psychiatrist, or who has a close loved one who may have this problem, reading this book is advised.

The DSM V states the following about Borderline Personality Disorder: a pervasive pattern of instability of interpersonal relationships, self image, and affects, and marked impulsivity, beginning by early adulthood and present in a variety of contexts as indicated by five or more of the following:

* *Frantic efforts to avoid real or imagined abandonment.*

* *A pattern of unstable and intense interpersonal relationships characterized by alternating extremes of idealization and devaluation. (My interpretation — you're either the best psychiatrist in the world or the worst. There are very few shades of gray in judging other people.)*

* *Identity disturbance: markedly and persistently unstable self-image or sense of self.*

* *Impulsivity in at least two areas that are potentially self-damaging (e.g. spending, sex, substance abuse, reckless driving, binge eating).*

* *Recurrent suicidal behavior, gestures, or threats, or self mutilating behavior.*

* *Affective instability due to marked reactivity of mood (e.g. intense episodic dysphoria, irritability, or anxiety usually lasting a few hours and only rarely more than a few days) depending on the happenings of that day especially with reference to interpersonal relations.*

* *Chronic feelings of emptiness.*

* *Inappropriate, intense anger or difficulty controlling anger (e.g. frequent displays of temper, constant anger, recurrent physical fights).*

* *Transient, stress-related paranoid ideation or severe dissociative symptoms.*

Dr. Paris emphasizes affective instability and impulsivity above everything else in his description of the borderline personality disorder. For practical purposes, I believe that if the psychiatrist can minimize the affective instability, this will also minimize the impulsivity. Any five or all of the nine descriptions by the DSM V can be present. The DSM V states that five of the above characteristics must be present to make the diagnosis. But for me, affective instability stands out above everything, and I am sure that I was influenced in this viewpoint by the writings of Dr. Paris. Dr. Paris points out that from a pharmacological viewpoint low doses of antipsychotic medications are the most effective at reducing affective instability. This is a "Pearl" as we say in medicine. Some of these patients will have severe persistent depression that requires an antidepressant in addition to a low-dose of an antipsychotic medication.

The origin of this problem is complex. Most of these patients experienced physical, sexual, or mental abuse during their childhood. I can usually find a history for this — usually. Sometimes parenting was inconsistent, lacking in guidance, neglectful. Children changing cultures are more prone to this problem than children who remain in the same culture until they are adults (from Dr. Paris — paraphrased).

Consequently, psychotherapy for this problem should probably be to some extent authoritarian setting guidelines and goals for behavior. Regressive types of psychotherapy, such as psychoanalysis, could possibly cause worsening of their symptoms. Cognitive Behavioral Therapy may be the preferred approach. Dr. Marsha M. Linehan has written extensively on this topic and even written workbooks as guidance for other mental health workers. She has also allowed comparisons of her outcomes in comparison to treatment as usual. She is well known as the originator of Dialectical Behavior Therapy.

Dr. Paris believes that one primary goal of psychotherapy should be competence in work performance of some type. He believes that competence in interpersonal relationships is a much more difficult goal to achieve. He also believes that the psychotherapy should focus more on problems here and now rather than traumas that occurred in the past.

Probably every type of psychotherapy has been utilized to treat borderline personality disorders. All therapists consider this extremely difficult. I have already made some statements about psychotherapy in the above paragraph. But, bottom line, the therapeutic alliance between the patient and the psychiatrist is probably more important than the type of psychotherapy (Luborsky, 1988). It stands to reason that paranoia, sometimes strong, could prevent any type of psychotherapy from occurring. The paranoid borderline personality disorder may come to therapy a few times, but shortly they will drop out of therapy due to their paranoia. They cannot trust the therapist.

Hospitalization is a must when they are extremely depressed and suicidal. Prolonged hospitalizations are unnecessary and may even allow non therapeutic regressive behavior. Their affect changes rapidly, so short hospitalizations may be all that is needed to prevent suicide. They will usually tell you, with a smile, when they are ready to be discharged. Sometimes partial hospitalization might be appropriate.

With frequent suicidal ideation or suicidal threats, you can understand the emotional stress this places on the therapist. He never knows when the patient will call with suicidal ideation — again. Some psychiatrists may find this to be more stressful than they can handle for their own emotional well-being. It is a major long-range commitment.

Sometimes the patient will need to be hospitalized repeatedly due to excessive self-mutilation such as cutting their wrist, or even their neck, shoulders, arms, chest, etc. An isolated incidence of self-mutilation may not require hospitalization, but repeated dangerous self-mutilation does require hospitalization. I knew one patient who would sneak a razor blade into the hospital in her shoe so that she could continue to self mutilate while in the hospital, causing the hospital personnel considerable angst.

Dr. Paris states that frequently suicide occurs when the patient loses hope, after failed therapeutic endeavors. Sometimes when a patient is uncooperative, the psychiatrist feels like "kicking back" and resting for a while, perhaps giving the patient a sense of hopelessness. It is important for the psychiatrist to always be optimistic and upbeat with any psychiatric patient so as to maintain their hope for feeling better. Even if he refers the patient to a different psychiatrist, if agreeable to the patient, this maintains the patient's hope for getting better. The patient's hope for getting better is very important no matter what the illness may be. Approximately 8 to 10 percent of these patients with borderline personality disorder will commit suicide.

Dr. Paris points out that the incidence of borderline personality disorder in our society is approximately 1.6 to

5.9 percent. This personality disorder may be present, to a greater or lesser extent, in patients who also have major depression or bipolar disorder or ADHD, etc. Fortunately this illness of affective instability, impulsivity, and problematic interpersonal relationships improves with age. Usually the 30s are better than the 20s. And usually the 40s are a time of marked improvement.

The DSM V has a few vignettes about patients to help the reader better understand this illness. And Dr. Paris gives 14 vignettes to help the reader better understand this illness. One patient, with whom I thought I had an excellent relationship, left a message stuck under a wad of gum on my office door indicating that I had deserted her, and she was furious with me. I was about 10 minutes late, at the most, due to hospital responsibilities and driving time between the two locations. Before that I had not recognized that she had these fears of abandonment.

In my experience, the patient may begin the relationship with subtle complements as to my abilities. At that point I become slightly uncomfortable because soon the patient will be expecting results I cannot deliver in a short period of time. As I stated earlier, you can be the best psychiatrist they have ever known, but soon you may be the worst they have ever known.

They sometimes cause "splitting" between health workers when they can. I find it difficult to describe how this is done; it can be quite subtle. They may tell their family physician that I blamed their headaches on some medication that he had prescribed; in reality, the patient told me that the medication had caused his headaches. Then I suggested that he should talk to his family physician about this.

The movie "Fatal Attraction" with Glenn Close and Michael Douglas might be considered an example of an extreme borderline personality disorder who would be willing to commit murder rather than lose the object of her affection. This is an extreme example, but it was a very entertaining movie.

Chapter 11

MARIJUANA

"Loyalty to a petrified opinion never yet broke a chain or freed a human soul." ~Mark Twain

I have never seen a marijuana cigarette. I have never smoked marijuana. To the best of my knowledge, I have never ingested any in a brownie. But I would like to tell you what hundreds of patients have told me about marijuana over the last 40 years. They told me all the usual things about improving appetite, greater appreciation of music, increased sensual feelings, euphoria, etc. I heard about this from the surfers in Southern California in the 1960s and 1970s. I am not here to extol the value of marijuana for getting "high." But I am here to let you know about the possible medicinal properties of marijuana for certain emotional miseries. And I will express a few opinions about the legalization of marijuana.

One of my patients was using marijuana to control panic attacks and generalized anxiety disorder. We both knew he was running a great risk of going to prison in the state of Louisiana (several years ago). He promised he would not smoke any more marijuana if I would give him some Xanax to cope with his panic attacks. But I was working for an organization at that time that would not allow me to give him any benzodiazepine. He told me that he would just have to keep using marijuana to cope with his miseries, running the risk of imprisonment. I was sad about this, but under the circumstances at that time, I had nothing to offer him in the way of a legal drug to replace his illegal drug. I never saw him again. The essence of the story is that many people use marijuana to control anxiety and panic attacks. In desperation, they are forced to repeatedly take serious risk to obtain it.

A great many patients, too numerous to count, have used marijuana or alcohol to slow their "racing mind" typical of mania. This is how many people become addicted to alcohol or marijuana. This is more likely to happen with younger manic patients. With age many of them join Alcoholics Anonymous and stop using alcohol. I do not think they have the classical "addictive personality" that psychiatrists frequently talk about. If they are simultaneously depressed (mixed mania), it is a major cause for suicide, perhaps the most frequent cause. They can never get over two to four hours of sleep on any night. They cannot focus on what they're doing. Marijuana may offer them some relief.

These patients tell me, when I ask, that marijuana is

more effective than alcohol to slow their racing mind. But many will use alcohol rather than marijuana because alcohol is legal, even if used in excess. Of course, as their tolerance grows, they will have to drink more and more alcohol to slow their "racing mind" leading to psychological and physical dependence. One patient who uses marijuana also told me that they have to use more and more marijuana as their tolerance grows with the passage of time; but withdrawal from marijuana is quite easy compared to withdrawal from alcohol. They may avoid marijuana for a few weeks; then when they use it again, it is effective in slowing their mind. But other patients have told me that they do not develop tolerance to the beneficial effects of marijuana. The bottom line to this paragraph is that marijuana may have some medicinal uses for the treatment of emotional and mental miseries such as "mixed mania."

I use antipsychotic medications, mood stabilizers, benzodiazepines, and sleep sedatives to slow their "racing mind." Are my medications as effective as marijuana for this purpose? Are my medications less deleterious to the central nervous system compared to marijuana? How does marijuana compare in cost to what I prescribe for my patients? I do not know. I know that what I do is legal. I know that what I do is much better for the racing mind than alcohol which is definitely neurotoxic. Marijuana may be less toxic to the central nervous system than alcohol. I do not mean that marijuana smoked in excess, about 10 joints per day, will not lead to changes in the brain; research shows that it will. I only mean to say that it might be less damaging to the brain when used at a maximum rate of two or three joints per day than alcohol.

Much research has been done concerning the effects of marijuana on the brain. Much of it comes from foreign countries because The National Institute of Drug Abuse (NIDA) limits the amount of research done in the United States by controlling the supply and quality of marijuana coming from the University of Mississippi, the only legal source in the United States. The U.S. Office of National Drug Control Policy has power over NIDA and NIDA has control over the FDA.

If we legalize marijuana, we will have one more mind altering substance to use, in addition to alcohol, to get "high." What is getting "high?" It is not the purpose of this chapter to do a scholarly discussion of getting "high." Most of you know what it is, as personally experienced. Many people who use a drug to get "high" will become psychologically and physically dependent on it (addicted). But most of us can have a drink on Friday night and maybe a drink on Saturday night also, and not get addicted. This is often referred to as "recreational" use of marijuana rather than "medicinal."

Sometimes what appears to be "recreational" use may in actuality be "medicinal" use. You and I do not know what demons that person may be contending with in his mind. But all we see on television concerning Colorado are these youthful people dressed in a somewhat antisocial manner taking a big puff of smoke from a marijuana cigarette and blowing it directly into the camera in defiance of "normal" society. But usually people drinking alcohol are portrayed as successful members of "normal" society. Television coverage shows the public what they want to see. Many people smoking marijuana in Colorado are not so youthful and would appear to be "normal" members of society. They simply prefer marijuana to alcohol.

I believe, as many people do, that marijuana has some medicinal uses to help cancer patients endure pain and reduce nausea and vomiting caused by chemotherapy, etc. Perhaps, with further investigation, marijuana might have some medicinal properties for certain psychiatric illnesses. Many of my patients thinks it does. Some of my psychiatric patients who are also in treatment for severe chronic pain tell me that marijuana relieves their pain as effectively as the narcotics they receive from their physician.

Some veterans with severe PTSD tell me that marijuana is more beneficial for relieving their symptoms of PTSD than any legal medication.

I just saw a TV program sponsored by PBS in which a man shrouded in darkness so that he could not be identified stated that he has taken every medication known to the medical profession to treat the pain and suffering caused by his Crohn's disease, a horrible illness affecting the lining of the small intestine. He had had 13 surgeries on his small intestine. A few puffs of marijuana would do much more for him than all of the medications and surgeries offered by the medical profession.

Recently I have heard on CNN about certain chemicals in marijuana controlling rare seizures that nothing else would control. I hear that it lowers intraocular pressure in glaucoma. Of course pharmaceutical companies will eventually discover medications derived from marijuana, to do these same things. And it will of course take a prescription from a medical doctor to obtain it. Many medicines need to be prescribed by a knowledgeable physician because they are dangerous. Marijuana is not dangerous in the hands of any reasonable person, and really does not need to be prescribed by a physician.

According to some research marijuana is not as dangerous to your health as nicotine. Nicotine has been legal since the beginning of this country. Please be sure to read "Effects of Cannabis" from Wikipedia, the free encyclopedia. Wikipedia analyzes 102 pieces of research on this topic. If you read this online, you can then go to each of the 102 pieces of research, click on them with your cursor, and read at least a summary of the research that they are basing their findings on. This topic is so controversial that is difficult to find research that is not biased by the beliefs or purposes of the researchers themselves.

The National Institute of Drug Abuse, the American Medical Association, and The American Psychiatric Association are all against the legalization of marijuana. One argument is that more research needs to be done concerning the effects of marijuana on the human brain. Of course more research would be better. But at this time I believe the research concerning marijuana is equivalent to the research done on most medications.

Other reasons for legalizing marijuana are well known to all of you. I wonder how many taxes could be collected with the legal sale of marijuana? I wonder how many people would be released from prison? I wonder how much taxpayer money could be saved by releasing these people from prison? Many of the prison beds in the United States are filled by people who are convicted of possession of a small amount of marijuana. Do you realize that private corporations, paid by the government to run these prisons, make a lot of money based on the number of prisoners they house?

We need those beds to house dangerous criminals. I wonder whether this would cut down on the thousands of murders annually, of each other, by people involved in the very profitable sale of illegal marijuana? I recently heard estimates on television that 80,000 people have been murdered in Mexico because of the illegal trafficking of marijuana since 1996. Remember, I am not arguing that you or anyone else should use marijuana. An argument for the legalization of marijuana is not an argument for using it. Those are two different topics. If you are a moral human being, enlarge your vision to look at this whole picture. Think about those people in prison. Think about those people murdered in Mexico. I have read that the annual murder rate in Guatemala is about 40 per hundred thousand people, 90 in Nicaragua, 45 in Venezuela, etc. These three countries are heavily involved in drug trafficking. By comparison the annual murder rate in the United States is less than 5 per hundred thousand people. The big bucks coming from North America are partially responsible for this. Every time someone buys illegal drugs, they should think about where their money is going.

I have heard, going back into the 1960s, about people using marijuana extensively and becoming very passive "dropouts" from society, abandoning productive work, etc. This has been a concern of mine with reference to chronic use of marijuana. This could be referred to as "Amotivational Syndrome." Something similar does occur with some chronic alcoholics, although this is not discussed very often. Some research concerning "Amotivational Syndrome" is included in Wikipedia. The conclusion of the authors of this paper is that amotivational syndrome could be a myth. It is certainly not well-founded on solid research. The authors speculate that these people who are lacking in motivation may be chronically intoxicated by cannabis, as some people will be.

Some people will not use marijuana at all. Some people will use it once or twice per week. Some people will use it once or twice daily. Some people will use it at the rate of 10 joints per day and be chronically intoxicated. But keeping marijuana illegal has not prevented this. "The World Drug Report" published in 2006 (a little old) showed that 162 million people in the world would try marijuana in a year's time; 75 million will use it less than one time per month; 66 million will use it two or three times weekly, and about 15 million will use it daily. Of that 15 million, about 7 million will stay chronically intoxicated (that is about four percent).

The North American market is estimated at somewhere between 10 and 60 billion dollars annually. North America is the number one market in the world, in spite of the drug being illegal. Most of the money goes to the smugglers, very little to the growers.

The United Nations "Global Drug Report" released in 2012, estimates that in the United States 28 percent of people age 18 to 25 use marijuana to some extent and 33 percent of children, seniors in high school, use marijuana to some extent.

Keeping it illegal is not preventing its use. The smugglers are making billions of dollars. They will spend big bucks to keep it illegal. I feel sure that the liquor industry would not want to see marijuana legalized. And even the pharmaceutical industry would not profit from the legalization of marijuana. Have you read about the massive amounts of money spent by the opposing sides when marijuana was legalized in Colorado?

One last thought about marijuana. Over and over my patients tell me about being beaten, screamed at, and even sexually molested by a father who was under the influence of alcohol. Some of them even told me that their father was a wonderful person when he was not intoxicated. I have never heard about anyone becoming physically violent under the influence of marijuana.

The research concerning marijuana, contained in Wikipedia and many other sources, is very extensive. But most Americans have not read this research, or even perused it. Overall, the discussion of this topic in our news media is very superficial. It is a hot topic that very few people in the news media are willing to discuss intelligently. The average American knows very little of the research concerning marijuana.

Research reveals that some people can become anxious and even paranoid under the influence of marijuana. I have seen a few schizophrenic patients, fairly stable, use marijuana and become paranoid and psychotic necessitating readmission to a psychiatric inpatient unit. I do not believe this is frequent in normal people, but some people can become anxious and paranoid under the influence of marijuana. And likewise, a few people can become psychotic under the influence of alcohol. I am sure those people will avoid using marijuana in the future after having had such a bad experience.

Recent research, quoted by NIDA and others, shows that between the ages of 13 and 38 approximately, daily use will result in an average drop in IQ of eight points. NIDA gives the impression that this research is based on psychological testing of 1037 people in New Zealand. Actually the researchers could find only 40 or 50 people out of 1037 who continued to use marijuana extensively from the ages of 13 to 38. Psychological testing was extensive and started well before the age of 13. The group reported these findings to the Proceedings of the National Academy of Science here in the United States. You can find details of this research on the NIDA website. This research did not show any change in memory if the smoker started during adult years.

There is a question about marijuana having a negative influence on brain development in young teenage children. Our society does not allow the use of alcohol before age 18, and I am sure that if marijuana were legalized, young people under 18 years of age could not legally use it. The use of marijuana under the age of 18 is rampant in this country at this time anyway. Most people believe that if it is legalized, more young people will use it. Certain young people are going to use mind altering substances more than other young people. Being legal or illegal does not altogether determine this. In fact, if young people think marijuana should be legal, they may use it even more in rebellion against their society.

An argument is frequently made that marijuana is a gateway substance to "harder drugs." My common sense tells me that if you have to obtain it from an illegal dealer that is also selling "harder drugs," you might be enticed by him to try "harder drugs." Legalizing marijuana would definitely diminish this possibility. You would not have to obtain it from an illegal dealer. And if legal, perhaps it would not be laced with cocaine or some other dangerous drug.

In a way, any mind altering substance is a gateway drug to other mind altering substances. This would definitely include alcohol. I had a patient who had just finished one month of rehabilitation trying to stop using cocaine. Immediately upon discharge from the hospital, he had gone home and drank a glass of wine in celebration of his wife's birthday. Under the influence of a little wine, he felt better about himself, more competent in all affairs including the possibility that he could use cocaine moderately. So he tried again to use cocaine moderately. He was not able to do so. I think any mind altering substance is a gateway to possibly using other mind altering substances. This would be true of alcohol also.

I am very frightened of cocaine, methamphetamine, and narcotics such as heroin or prescribed narcotics. I do not have the courage to experiment even once with any one of them. I have been told that some people can use cocaine moderately without destroying themselves. But in my practice of medicine, I have never met one of these people. The people I work with are always trying to stop, but often failing. I have known too many women who would prostitute themselves to obtain cocaine. I once knew a woman who prostituted her young daughter, age 12 or 13, to obtain cocaine. I have known men who have committed robberies to obtain cocaine. I am very frightened of the addictive potential of these drugs.

I have known people so addicted to heroin that they were also addicted to the stick of the needle and the injection of the liquid. When they cannot obtain heroin, they will take a needle and syringe and inject water or normal saline into their vein anyway. The needlestick is associated with increased dopamine which causes a "high" to a degree because the needlestick is always associated in their mind with the high obtained from heroin. The National Institute of Drug Abuse (NIDA) tells me that heroin and certain other narcotics are the very hardest of all addictions to break. When addicts stop these narcotics, they experience a depression from hell. This is also true when cocaine and methamphetamine addicts attempt to stop. The physical withdrawal is a small problem, comparatively speaking. The psychological withdrawal is the only real problem. The depression gets better with time, but it can last for years.

Narcotic addicts frequently die within a few years. That is why the federal government allows certain physicians to prescribe Suboxone sublingually to help them live into the future. They can take it for several years, or longer, if necessary to avoid using illegal narcotics. Suboxone is itself a narcotic, but it is safer to take long-term than the illegal narcotics. The federal government also allows methadone clinics to help people stop using heroin and other narcotics. Methadone is a narcotic also. The federal government recognizes the horrible grip that narcotics have on these addicts. They simply cannot stop taking it.

These drugs all cause more dopamine in the brain; unfortunately, the brain responds by reducing the number of dopamine receptors, which cause pleasure. This is what causes the depression from hell. And the addict has to keep taking more and more of his drug of choice to avoid this depression from hell. NIDA (National Institute on Drug Abuse) has been a major source of knowledge for me on this topic.

Like alcohol, someone under the influence of marijuana would be more likely to have a traffic accident due to impaired coordination or judgment. There would have to be laws curtailing driving under the influence of alcohol and marijuana. Currently urine drug screens reveal if a person has used marijuana during the last month, and not whether they are currently under the influence. But there are sophisticated tests that will show the current blood level of marijuana. This would solve the problem. It is usually reported in nanograms/milliliters.

Synthetic marijuana, currently becoming popular because it does not show up in a drug screen, is much more damaging to the brain than marijuana. If marijuana were legalized, hopefully people would quit using synthetic marijuana.

It will be easier to overdose with marijuana ingesting it orally rather than smoking it. The effects of smoking are felt much sooner. It is just easier to overdose orally than it is by smoking. Overdosage has definite bad effects psychologically. It can cause severe anxiety and even psychosis. It will increase the heart rate significantly. If the user has underlying heart disease, this might lead to death.

Smoking will cause bronchitis. Vaporizing may avoid bronchitis. The research to date shows it to be less likely to cause cancer of the lungs than tobacco, but I cannot know what future research will reveal.

Addendum: Just as I finished writing this chapter, my wife, in the Atlanta airport, found a copy of "The Gazette," a newspaper serving the Colorado Springs and Pikes Peak region since 1872 that won the 2014 Pulitzer Prize for national reporting. The name of the article is "Pioneer in Pot" by Carol McGraw and Megan Schrader. They detail multiple organizations and individuals that donated money to bring about legalization of pot in Colorado. It amazed me as to the number of organizations all over this country that came together to bring this about. Certain individuals donated large sums of money to this cause. Certain organizations were opposed, but they were far outspent by the organizations in favor. The article details the vote count in various counties of the state. Certain counties will not allow it to be sold in that county. The current law in Colorado says which agency regulates the sale of marijuana, who can buy (over age 21), who can grow at home and how much, where you can't partake in public, penalties, etc. Anyone driving under the influence of more than 5 ng/ml in their blood would be subject to legal penalties. Also there are limits as to how much an individual can possess in the solid or liquid form at any time. Some of the penalties are fairly severe. But the summary of all of the organizations that came together to legalize pot in Colorado is astounding. It was quite a political battle. The reporting by Carol McGraw and Megan Schrader in "The Gazette" is excellent, in my opinion. This edition was published on Sunday, April 27, 2014 (www.gazette.com).

Addendum #2: It is now 2019. I originally finished writing this book in 2015. I would like to add some information to the original chapter on Marijuana.

Everyone knows about anandamides today. Four or five years ago I thought this would be too technical for this small book. In a nutshell, the receptors in the brain and the gut for some of the marijuana chemicals are originally designated by the body for receptors of a neurotransmitter called anandamide. This is a little beyond my scope of knowledge in that there were at least 27 chemicals found in the marijuana plant five years ago. I would imagine that they have now discovered even more chemicals in this one plant. The receptors in the brain are named CBT 1 receptors, even though they were originally anandamide receptors. The receptors in the lower intestine are called CBT 2 receptors. I told you earlier about the man shrouded in darkness on television talking about the best relief from pain, due to Crohn's disease in his small intestine being due to smoking marijuana. There is research to show that people smoking marijuana are about 30% less likely to overdose with the narcotics they are using, prescribed by their physician, for chronic pain. Severe chronic pain is one cause of suicide. Marijuana used in conjunction with a narcotic, if absolutely necessary, for severe chronic pain is more effective than narcotics alone. Ideally, I would rather see the patient using marijuana alone when possible because the narcotics or so addictive for some people.

Some of my patients knew early on that they should not use narcotics for pain. They knew that they "like them too much." People addicted to alcohol have told me that they were addicted after the first drink. These two statements are the exception, not the rule, but narcotics can be more addictive for some people than others. And narcotics are much more dangerous in overdosage by far than marijuana.

Everyone knows about cannabidiol now. It is one of the 27 chemicals in the marijuana plant. It can also be extracted from the hemp plant originally used in the 13 colonies to make rope. There are several ways to perform this extraction. What you want is cannabidiol in the purest form possible with the least amount of impurities. But one lecturer on this topic told me that one form of extraction brings certain chemicals out with the cannabidiol which make it even more effective in relieving pain. This mixture is superficially referred to as extract. Essentially, I know nothing about these various methods of extraction. I hope my reader will obtain information from other sources about this. The cannabidiol or cannabidiol extract contained no THC. As you know, this part of marijuana is becoming legal in many states with attached provisions. It is useful in many illnesses including arthritic pain. It may actually affect the immune system in a beneficial manner (purely conjecture on my part).

In 2015 at the American Psychiatric Association

annual meeting in Toronto, a brilliant young neurologist and immunologist, affiliated with Harvard and the Dana Farber Cancer Institute, presented research showing that marijuana caused an increase in the CD4 count of patients being treated for HIV. So I have some reason for thinking that marijuana may actually affect the immune system in a positive way. Her name was Dr. Gabuzda.

I met a young woman in 2015 coming home on a plane from Toronto. I gave her a copy of my new book just published. Within the next week or so, I received an email from her telling me how much she appreciated the chapter on marijuana. Her father had bipolar illness. He probably did not realize what his problem was. The only relief he obtained from his racing mind and insomnia was marijuana. It was very illegal at that time. He ended his life by suicide.

Addendum #3: This is the third edition of this book. My experience with marijuana users was between 1994 and 2017. Before 1990 the typical THC concentration in marijuana was less than 5%. Now there are many plants being cultivated containing 17 to 28% THC. Each marijuana product for sale has its own name. I found quite easily on THEWEEDBLOG 19 different names for these products. For use medically, as the concentration of

THC increases, the concentration of CBD decreases. I originally thought that CBD alone would be the preferred use for medicinal purposes. Later I came to know that the CBD extract containing certain terpenes and perhaps other chemicals was more therapeutic than CBD alone. More recently, I have been told by people prescribing marijuana for medicinal purposes that some amount of THC in addition to CBD extract was more beneficial for medicinal purposes. I do not know the exact amount of THC that should be included, and I think there would be several different opinions at this point in time as to the exact amount of THC that should be present in medicinal marijuana.

Withdrawal from marijuana containing less than 5% THC was fairly easy, so my patients told me. I am now speculating that withdrawal from these higher concentrations of THC could produce a fairly serious, or maybe very serious depression. Still speculating, if THC, a stimulant like cocaine for example, causes a decrease in dopamine receptors like cocaine does (information from NIDA) then a prolonged and serious depression might follow. All of the feel-good drugs like cocaine cause more dopamine at the receptor sites. The brain responds by decreasing the number of dopamine receptors. As we all know, the cocaine user must constantly increase the dose to get the "high" he got from the first time he used it. Since these dopamine receptors are essential for any of us to have feelings of happiness or well-being, you can imagine the depression a cocaine user experiences when he stops cocaine which causes high levels of dopamine. No receptors—no pleasures. Might something like this occur when the individual stops using the marijuana containing high percentage of THC? Other mental health workers will have to question the users of high THC as to the severity of withdrawal symptoms.

Now a concentrated form of THC is being extracted from crushed marijuana. The concentration varies from 40 to 80% THC. This concentrate has many street names. Two of them are "honey" and "budder." This concentrate is usually obtained through water pipes or oil pipes. It has caused mental changes to paranoia, anxiety, panic attacks, hallucinations, etc.

This area of knowledge is changing so rapidly that perhaps I should not have included it in this book. But several people who liked my original book were most thankful for the chapter on marijuana. They had themselves or relatives who had relieved miseries caused by various forms of mania, with the racing mind and insomnia. At that time, marijuana was unlawful all over the United States. Marijuana will not cure even mild states of mania. It only helped to a degree. I should point out at this time that bipolar disorder and mania can vary from extremely severe with multiple hospitalizations to very mild with no hospitalizations and sometimes not even medication.

Chapter 12

INSOMNIA

Insomnia accompanies almost all mental health ill-nesses. Insomnia is also a problem associated with many neurological illnesses such as ADHD, narcolepsy, restless leg syndrome, etc. Insomnia is also associated with an anatomical problem called obstructive sleep apnea. I will be discussing insomnia only as a complication of mental health illnesses and certain neurological illnesses.

A small percentage of the medical profession under-estimates the importance of insomnia, and the importance of treating insomnia. Perhaps they are afraid to give a con-trolled medications such as a benzodiazepine for relief. This is lacking in empathy and lacking in understanding of the importance of treating insomnia. Fortunately this is only a small part of the medical profession. There is a movement in progress in the medical profession prompt-ing all physicians to treat chronic pain appropriately. I think there should be a movement in the medical pro-fession to treat insomnia appropriately. It is impossible to treat mental illnesses effectively without also treating the insomnia that accompanies these mental illnesses. And some people have insomnia for completely unknown causes. They need treatment also.

People with bipolar disorder who are in a manic state cannot fall asleep for 2 to 4 hours, and maybe even longer. People with bipolar disorder in remission can be pushed into a manic state by missing several nights of sleep.

People with generalized anxiety disorder or depression may be miserable due to early-morning awakening. If they get only five or six hours of sleep, they will be fatigued all day long.

People with narcolepsy, a neurological illness, only reach light REM sleep. They never reach deep, restorative Non-Rem(NREM) sleep. Consequently they are famous for taking short naps all through the day.

Difficulty falling asleep may be a complication of ADHD, but fortunately it is not always a complicating factor in ADHD.

Some people who drink alcohol fall asleep easily, but may awake at 1 AM or 2 AM with their mind racing and stimulated. This is sometimes referred to as rebound insomnia. They will be very fatigued the following day.

Many schizophrenic patients who are feeling good can stop their medication and become agitated. Their relatives will report that they are "pacing the floor" all night long. I have heard this story repeatedly concerning schizophrenic patients who are being readmitted to a psychiatric unit.

People under severe stress of any kind may have difficulty sleeping.

Some research shows that insomnia may be a major factor in the etiology of Alzheimer's Disease, heart disease, obesity, diabetes, alcohol use, and hypertension.

If you go to a physician seeking help for any form of insomnia, he may talk to you first about sleep hygiene. All of the available medications have mild to moderate complications associated with them. The rules of sleep hygiene sound rather simple, but they are not as simple as they sound. Some people will not be able to take any form of caffeine, even including chocolates, after 2 PM. Some people cannot even drink a single cup of coffee in the morning. Other people can drink several cups of coffee spread out through their daytime hours. Other people can drink a cup of coffee at 10 PM and be asleep by 10:30 PM. Some people cannot exercise just before bedtime, but other people will find this helps them to sleep. Exercise in general might be the best treatment for insomnia for many people. Some people should only use the bed for sleeping or intimacy. But other people can only fall asleep in the bed if they are watching something on television. They cannot fall asleep if it is completely quiet in the room. Sleep hygiene dictates that you do not lie in bed much longer than 20 minutes trying to fall asleep. This is a miserable situation, and sleep hygiene would advise you to get up and watch television or read until you get sleepy enough to fall asleep. Sleep hygiene advises you to diminish the stress in your life.

Personally, diminishing the stress in my life is my best treatment for my own insomnia. And exercise is very important for me, especially as I get older and have more problems with insomnia. But sometimes it is very difficult to find a way to diminish stress. And many of my patients cannot exercise very much due to multiple physical disabilities. Remember, exercise is a privilege, not a burden. Most disabled people will remind you of that fact.

Some people are just more prone to anxiety than others; they may be diagnosed as clinically depressed or having a generalized anxiety disorder. They will tend to be able to go to sleep, but their problem will be early-morning awakening after having obtained only five or six hours of sleep. They will probably be fatigued all day long. Maybe some form of psychotherapy or meditation could help them to fall asleep. But after doing everything we can to sleep without using medications, medications may be needed to treat insomnia. But medications with potential side effects should obviously be the last choice.

For a few people alcohol might seem to be a good sleep medication. They may have a couple of jiggers and sleep all night. Most people would have a rebound insomnia awakening just a few hours after going to sleep. That is why one of the usual recommendations for sleep hygiene is to avoid alcohol before bedtime. Those people who sleep well following alcohol ingestion may need to take larger and larger amounts with the passage of time. This is an expensive sleep medication, and the withdrawal can be quite severe. I would never recommend alcohol as a sleep medication.

The neurotransmitter histamine keeps us awake during the daytime. The neurotransmitter GABA (gamma amino butyric acid) slows neurotransmission in the brain and helps us to go to sleep. So all of the sleep medications either suppress histamine (anti-histaminic) or enhance the GABA receptors to slow neurotransmission in the brain.

The drugs that enhance the GABA receptors are the Z drugs like Ambien (zolpidem), Lunesta (eszoplicone), or Sonata (Zaleplon). Benzodiazepines like Valium (diazepam), Ativan (lorazepam), Xanax (alprazolam), Restoril (temazepam), etc. also enhance the GABA receptors. Many physicians are more comfortable prescribing a medication that has anti-histaminic properties rather than a controlled substance medication that enhances the GABA receptors. I have talked about this in my chapter "Addressing the Prejudice Against Benzodiazepines."

The classic antihistamine would be Benadryl (diphenhydramine). Most of the antihistaminic medications have anticholinergic effects also. This is the major drawback of these medications. Anti-cholinergic means to suppress acetylcholine throughout the body. Acetylcholine is important for thinking, constriction of the pupil, movement of the gut, slowing of the heart, etc. For some people the anticholinergic side effects of Benadryl are minimal, and it is a good sleep medication. Other people will be constipated, "hung over" the next day, etc. due to the anticholinergic side effects. But Benadryl overall is a good sleep medication for many people.

Some of the drugs used for their antihistaminic properties have more serious side effects. For example, an old tricyclic antidepressant Elavil (amitriptyline) can cause severe cardiac dysrhythmias if taken in overdosage, which is always a possibility for people with emotional miseries. It also causes increased appetite, weight gain, etc. Seroquel (quetiapine) an antipsychotic medication has strong antihistaminic properties, but it can cause weight gain, adult onset diabetes, increased cholesterol, postural hypotension, etc. So I think that the medications with antihistaminic properties are just as dangerous as the controlled substances that enhance the GABA receptors. Except for Benadryl, I feel it is better for the patient to use a controlled substance that enhances the GABA receptors rather than most of the antihistaminic drugs mentioned above.

The side effects of the Z drugs and benzodiazepines are less usually. Ambien (zolpidem) can cause sleepwalking which is sometimes dangerous. This is a small percentage of patients, but it can be alarming when it happens. One in 25 patients, or less, cannot metabolize Valium (diaz-epam) normally. They do not have certain liver enzymes that the vast majority of people have. Consequently the first dose they take might cause them to sleep for two or three days. Klonopin (clonazepam) can rarely cause ataxia. The patient will feel as if they are "drunk." Proper warning of the patient about these rare side effects can prevent disasters from occurring. In overdosage, they do not stop respiration and kill people unless they are mixed with alcohol, narcotics, or some other sedative drug. One emergency room physician told me that he could easily handle a patient overdosed with benzodiazepines in com-parison to a patient overdosed with some of the above described antihistaminic substances. Flumazenil, given intravenously, can briefly reverse the effects of overdosage of a benzodiazepine. It has to be given several times at certain time intervals to maintain this reversal. But there are a few patients with an "addictive personality" who can-not take benzodiazepines appropriately.

The Z drugs (Ambien, Lunesta, and Sonata) attach only to the GABA a 1 receptors. They promote sleep, but they do very little if anything for anxiety. The benzodiaze-pines attached to GABA a 1, 2,3,5 receptors and are very effective for anxiety and promoting sleep. But physical dependence does develop with any of these drugs.

And I should point out in passing that none of these drugs alone will promote sleep if someone is in a state of mania. Instead of using larger and larger doses of these sleep promoting medications, they will need mood stabilizers, antipsychotic medications etc. in addition to these sleep promoting drugs.

As far as physical dependence is concerned, some people can take a benzodiazepine for years and hardly notice the withdrawal. Other people will have severe withdrawal symptoms such as racing heart, rapid breathing, mental stimulation, severe inability to sleep. They may need professional help with these miseries.

Why worry about withdrawal? Why not just keep taking the effective medication? Well, the medication may become ineffective after three or four years. You cannot sleep with it, and you have withdrawal when you stop it. This can be more painful for the elderly who have less cardiac reserves etc. One could increase the dose, but then when the medicine ceases to be effective again, the withdrawal might be very severe. So I advise changing from one sleep medication to another sleep medication for a month or so. Then, after a period of time, the original medication will be effective again.

I advise everyone to use the least amount of medication that promotes adequate sleep. If stressors are diminished, they may be able to discontinue all sleep medication. Sometimes people find out that they can fall asleep without any sleep medication, but when they awaken about 2:30 are 3 AM, they need a small amount of sleep medication to get their needed eight hours of sleep. For many people 5mg of generic Ambien (which is less potent than brand name Ambien) will effect them for only three or four hours. I say this in spite of the fact that the FDA has recently put a Black Box Warning on Ambien that some women cannot metabolize it in eight hours and could have a traffic accident the next morning. The FDA advises women to take only 5 mg of Ambien, and it should be taken upon going to sleep, not after four or five hours of sleep. Each person has a different reaction to these sleep medications. They should be started very carefully, preferably on a weekend when they do not have to get up early the next morning. And caution needs to be exercised before driving a motor vehicle the next morning. But the major problem with Ambien is sleep walking, which can be dangerous. I have heard many stories from my patients about the dangerous things they did while sleep walking.

Without eight hours, some people will be fatigued all day long. The elderly may notice heart rhythm changes, joint aching, etc. due to lack of sleep. There is some recent research indicating that everyone who uses benzodiazepines for sleep has their life shortened. That research encouraged everyone to use cognitive behavioral therapy to solve their sleep problems. Well, I agree with this. But when improving sleep hygiene or some form of psychotherapy does not help, I believe using medication and getting adequate sleep will prolong their life, not shorten it. Without the use of sleep medication, their lives might have been shortened even more. Remember, insomnia may cause heart disease, Alzheimer's, obesity, diabetes, etc.

Very recently some research has indicated that the antihistaminic drugs, taken over a long period of time, could contribute to dementia. I cannot remember if it was earlier onset of dementia or more serious dementia? I have only seen one reference to this possibility.

And some fortunate people can use the same sleep medication successfully for 10 or 15 years without it losing its effectiveness. But I never know who that is in advance. Consequently, I always warn the patient about possible loss of effectiveness with time and possible withdrawal miseries. I never use sleep medication if the patient can sleep without it

Of course, the lucky people who do not experience insomnia to any great extent are probably the healthiest of us all. And they are very lucky if they do not experience insomnia with aging.

A very few medications enhance the functioning of GABA neurons to induce sleep by attaching to the GABA b receptors. Remember that the Z drugs and the benzodiazepines effect some of the six GABA a receptors, not the GABA b receptors. These drugs that affect the GABA b receptors promote deeper non-rem sleep. That would be exactly what the person with narcolepsy needs. As I mentioned earlier, these patients can never get deep sleep and consequently they take multiple naps during the day. Enhancement of the functioning of the GABA b receptors would be of great benefit in narcolepsy. One medication used for this purpose is Xyrem (sodium oxybate). It has also been called GHB (gamma hydroxy butyrate). Only physicians who have a certain amount of training in the use of this medication can prescribe. It is tightly controlled by the DEA because a few people have accidentally overdosed with it.

Why not just take more GABA for the treatment of insomnia? GABA will not cross the blood brain barrier. It could be given orally, by intramuscular injection, or any other way, but it cannot get to the brain. There is a medication called Phenibut that can reach the brain if taken orally. The chemical name is beta phenyl gamma amino butyric acid. This might be similar to taking more GABA. It was developed in the Soviet Union in the 1960s and is used for anxiety, PTSD, and insomnia. The more one reads about GABA, the more interesting the topic becomes. Phenibut is not available in the United States.

There is one more medication available for the treatment of insomnia. That medication is melatonin. Melatonin is available in health food stores without a prescription. Melatonin is released by the pineal gland and probably has it effects via the suprachiasmatic nucleus which functions as the brains internal clock, regulating the awake-sleep cycles. The pineal gland is sensitive to light and releases melatonin at night to exert its effect on the suprachiasmatic nucleus. Consequently histamine is no longer released to keep us awake. Thus melatonin induces sleep, but may not be effective in maintaining sleep throughout the night.

Many people will take 3 mg to 6 mg of melatonin orally to induce sleep. However, when taken sublingually (under the tongue), it will go straight to the blood stream, and only 0.5 mg or 1 mg can be as effective as 3 mg to 6 mg orally, theoretically. Most medications taken orally will go through the stomach to the liver, and the liver will metabolize a large portion of this foreign substance so that much of it does not reach the bloodstream or the brain. Many medications taken sublingually are more effective than if they were taken orally. But in my personal experience, some brands of melatonin are much stronger than others; consequently the brand may be more important than the route of administration. Some trial and error is probably needed to find a good brand of melatonin. Generic benzodiazepine brands vary as to strength also, no matter what the milligram dosage is supposed to be.

There is another medication called Rozerem (ramelton) that is a direct agonist on the melatonin receptors in the suprachiasmatic nucleus (brains internal clock). I'm not sure if Rozerem sensitizes these melatonin receptors to melatonin or is simply another form of melatonin? The result is the same. For some reason it will not have its effects until after 4 or 5 days of use. I have no experience with Rozerem.

To summarize, the treatment of insomnia is absolutely essential for the successful treatment of most mental health illnesses. All physicians should be aware of the importance of treating insomnia. But when possible, insomnia should be treated without the use of medication. Unfortunately, medication is often necessary and can be lifesaving.

I have not emphasized the importance of properly treating the underlying psychiatric illness, if any, before treating insomnia. Insomnia may or may not exist after treatment of the psychiatric illness.

Conclusion

In the future, possibly 10 years from now, more or less, the genetic scientist may help us to make diagnoses in psychiatry via genetic testing. Currently, it appears that several genes can be involved in the origin of any clinically diagnosed mental illness. Now, psychiatrist can send saliva specimens to certain laboratories which can tell you what medications the patient may respond to based on liver enzymes responsible for metabolism of these medications. It can be difficult to get a therapeutic level of a medication which that liver metabolizes very quickly. Also, a patient cannot take Valium (diazepam) if they do not have certain liver enzymes. Some genetic scientist believe that certain people are more prone to commit suicide than others. In other words, a very depressed patient may or may not be a serious suicidal risk in spite of their misery. I'm not sure that this is fully agreed upon by all genetic scientist. I've already mentioned in the chapter on "Depression" that some people, genetically speaking, are more prone to depression than others. Some genetic scientist believe that certain people following traumatic experiences are more prone to PTSD than other people. Genetic scientist pretty much agree that children with ADHD may have genetic tendencies to bipolar disorder, depression, anxiety, etc. ADHD is definitely a more serious mental problem in some cases than the general public is aware of. Others seem to "outgrow" this problem as they near adulthood. The general public is not aware that ADHD can be a serious problem throughout adult life.

As neuroscientist learn more and more, it is becoming gradually more and more difficult for me to understand what they are talking about. I could keep up, when explained, at first; but this is becoming harder and harder to understand or memorize. They are so specialized; I wonder if one neuroscientist working in one field can fully understand what a different neuroscientist working in another field is discovering.

Currently, diagnoses still have to be made primarily by clinical expertise. This is acquired by very carefully listening to our patients and trying to build on the knowledge that psychiatrist working over the last 100 years have gradually acquired. We are all indebted to those who came before us. But, Mark Twain commented that *"The problem is not what you do not know; the problem is what you do know that is not true."* In my opinion, in some cases, he was correct.